Rapid ECG
Interpretation

Rapid ECG
Interpretation

M. Gabriel Khan,
MD, FRCP (London), FRCP(C), FACP, FACC

Associate Professor of Medicine
University of Ottawa
Cardiologist, Ottawa General Hospital
Ottawa, Ontario
Canada

W.B. SAUNDERS COMPANY
A Division of Harcourt Brace & Company
Philadelphia   London   Toronto   Montreal   Sydney   Tokyo

W.B. SAUNDERS COMPANY

A Division of Harcourt Brace & Company

The Curtis Center
Independence Square West
Philadelphia, Pennsylvania 19106

Library of Congress Cataloging-in-Publication Data

Khan, M. I. Gabriel.
  Rapid ECG interpretation / M. Gabriel Khan.
      p.   cm.
  ISBN 0-7216-7468-2
  1. Electrocardiography.   I. Title.
  [DNLM: 1. Electrocardiography—handbooks.   WG 39 K45r 1997]
RC683.5.E5K48   1997
616.1'207547—dc21
DNLM/DLC
                                                              97-12030

RAPID ECG INTERPRETATION   ISBN 0-7216-7468-2

Printed in the United States of America

Last digit is the print number: 9   8   7   6   5   4   3   2

Preface

This text presents a unique 11-step method for rapid ECG interpretation in a user-friendly synopsis format. I developed this rapid, accurate method for interpretation of the ECG over a 24-year period while interpreting more than 200,000 ECGs and giving numerous seminars to medical students on ECG interpretation.

The method is based on sound cardiologic decision-making algorithms that can be computerized. In developing the method I raised the questions, How does a cardiologist arrive at an ECG diagnosis? What steps does the expert interpreter take in his mind as he interprets an ECG? Analysis of this scenario reveals that the essential steps are algorithms that are rapidly synchronized by the human brain. This method departs from the conventional approach—rate, rhythm, axis, hypertrophy—in that the diagnoses of infarction, ischemia, and rhythm disturbances, which are of paramount importance clinically, are placed early in the steps ahead of diagnosis of the axis. In interpreting 200 tracings weekly I find it makes more sense clinically to deal with the axis near the end of the interpretive sequence rather than early, as is taught in most textbooks.

The 11 steps are illustrated in algorithms and outlined in Chapter 1 with cross-references to later chapters, each of which expands on one of the steps. **All diagnostic ECG criteria are covered succinctly,** providing a quick review or refresher for cardiologists preparing for the American College of Cardiology ECG Proficiency Test and for physicians preparing for the ECG section of the Cardiovascular Diseases Board Examination.

Despite the advent of expensive and sophisticated cardiologic tests the ECG remains the most reliable tool for the confirmation of acute myocardial infarction. The ECG—not the CK-MB, echocardiogram, or SPECT or PET scan—dictates the rapid administration of lifesaving thrombolytic therapy. There is no test to rival the ECG in the diagnosis of arrhythmias, which is a common clinical cardiologic problem. Also, the diagnosis of pericarditis and myocardial ischemia can only be confirmed by ECG findings. This text can be a valuable tool for all those who wish to be proficient in the interpretation of ECGs.

M. GABRIEL KHAN

Acknowledgments

Richard Zorab, Senior Medical Editor, W.B. Saunders, had the good sense to foster the production of this book.

Joan Sinclair and Michele Garber of W.B. Saunders and Mary Espenschied deserve special mention.

I had the privilege of borrowing several ECG tracings from the fourth edition of Electrocardiography in Clinical Practice by the late Dr. Te-Chuan Chou and from Practical Electrocardiography by Dr. Henry J.L. Marriott. I am grateful to these authors, true masters of the art of ECG interpretation.

M. GABRIEL KHAN

Contents

CHAPTER 1

Method for Rapid ECG Interpretation **1**

CHAPTER 2

The P Wave **54**

CHAPTER 3

Genesis of the QRS Complex **59**

CHAPTER 4

Bundle Branch Block **64**

CHAPTER 5

ST Segment Abnormalities **74**

CHAPTER 6

Q Wave Abnormalities **98**

CHAPTER 7

Atrial and Ventricular Hypertrophy **136**

CHAPTER 8

T Waves **145**

CHAPTER 9

Electrical Axis and Fascicular Block **160**

CHAPTER 10

Miscellaneous Conditions **172**

CHAPTER 11

Arrhythmias **197**

1

Method for Rapid ECG Interpretation

Close attention to the 11 steps for rapid electrocardiogram (ECG) interpretation outlined in this chapter and reference to detailed explanations given in this and subsequent chapters should allow students, housestaff, and practicing clinicians to be competent interpreters of most ECGs. Rapid, but accurate, interpretation of the ECG requires a methodical approach.

Figure 1–1 defines the ECG wave form. Figure 1–2 shows normal ECG tracings. Table 1–1 lists important intervals and parameters. The ECG interpretation should end with one of the following statements:

- Normal ECG
- Within normal limits
- Borderline ECG
- Abnormal ECG

STEP 1: ASSESS RHYTHM AND RATE (Fig. 1–3)

Focus on leads V_1, V_2, and II (Fig. 1–2). Leads V_1 and II are best for visualization of P waves to determine the presence of sinus rhythm or an arrhythmia. V_1 and V_2 are best to observe for bundle branch block. If P waves are not clearly visible in V_1, assess them in lead II, which usually shows well-formed P waves. Identification of the P wave and then the RR intervals allows the interpreter to discover immediately whether the rhythm is sinus or other and to

- Confirm, if it is a sinus rhythm, that the RR intervals are equidistant (Fig. 1–2A), that the P wave is positive in lead II, and that the PP intervals are equidistant and equal to the RR interval.

Text continued on page 10

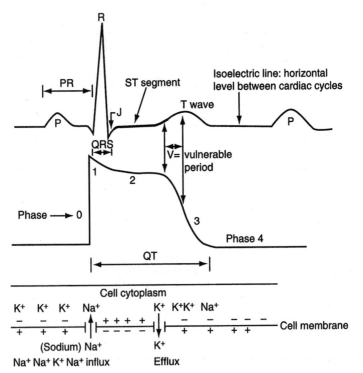

FIGURE 1–1   Sodium influx, potassium efflux, the action potential, and the electrocardiogram. (From Khan MG. On Call Cardiology. Philadelphia: WB Saunders, 1997, p 48.)

TABLE 1–1   *Important Normal ECG Intervals and Parameters**

PR interval	0.12 to 0.2 second (rarely up to 0.24 second).
P waves	< 3 small squares (0.12 second) in duration, and amplitude < 3 mm. Upright in lead I, inverted in aVR (if opposite, suspect reversed arm leads[†] or dextrocardia) (see step 6, Figs. 1–21 and 1–36).
QRS duration	0.04 to 0.1 second; > 0.1 second, consider LBBB, RBBB, or WPW syndrome (see steps 2 and 3, Figs. 1–4, 1–9, and 1–10).
Q waves	Normally present in aVR; occasionally in V_1 or in aVL (vertical heart) (see Chapter 6).
	Often present in lead III: should be ≤ 0.04 second duration and ≤ 7 mm deep.
	Other leads except lead I: < 0.04 second duration and ≤ 3 mm deep; lead I ≤ 1.5 mm over age 30. Q's may be up to 5 mm deep in several leads in individuals < age 30 (see p. 98).
R waves	V_1: 0 to 15 mm, age 12 to 20.
	0 to 8 mm, age 20 to 30.
	0 to 6 mm, age > 30[‡] (see p. 103).
	V_2: 0.2 to 12 mm, age > 30[†] (see step 5, Fig. 1–15).
	V_3: 1 to 20 mm, age > 30.[†]
ST segment	Isoelectric or < 1 mm elevation in limb leads; < 2 mm in precordial leads except for normal variant (see step 4, Fig. 1–12).
T wave	Inverted in aVR; upright in I, II, and V_3 through V_6.
	Variable in III, aVF, aVL, V_1, and V_2 (see step 8, Fig. 1–27).
Axis	0° to +110° age < 40.
	–30° to +90° age > 40 (see step 9, Fig. 1–30).
QT interval	See Table 1–5, page 47, and page 174.

*ECG paper speed 25 mm/s.
†Precordial leads remain normal.
‡Age > 30 is relevant to the diagnosis of myocardial infarction. See page 103, poor R wave progression.

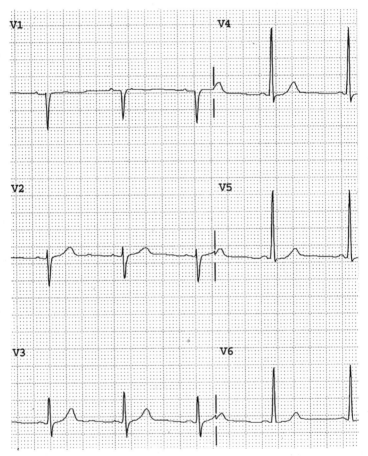

FIGURE 1–2   A, Chest leads V_1 through V_6.

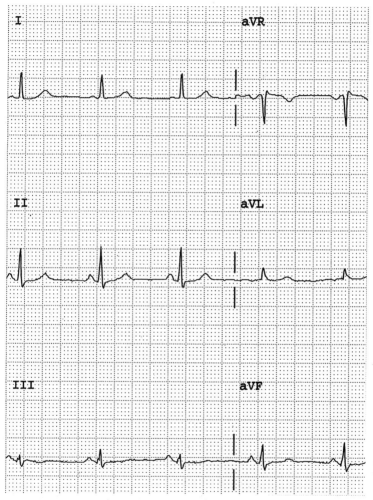

FIGURE 1–2 *Continued* **B,** Limb leads, I through aVF. Sinus rhythm, rate 65 beats per minute (bpm), PR interval 0.14 second, QRS duration 0.08 second, QT interval 0.36 second, axis +30°. Note normal small Q wave in V_4 through V_6.

Figure continued on following page

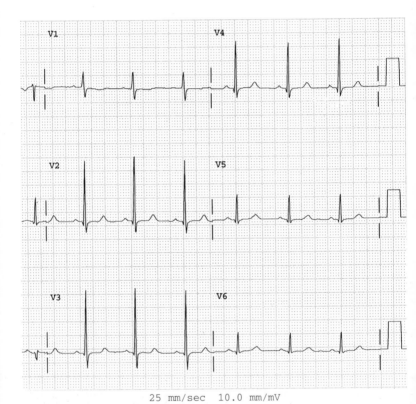

25 mm/sec   10.0 mm/mV

FIGURE 1–2 *Continued*   **C,** Chest leads of a normal ECG with a QRS complex in V$_2$ that is positive, indicating early transition. Compare with Figure 1–2*A* in which transition is normal, occurring in lead V$_3$; tall R waves in V$_1$ and V$_2$ are not caused by posterior infarction (Table 1–3). Heart rate 75 bpm (Table 1–2).

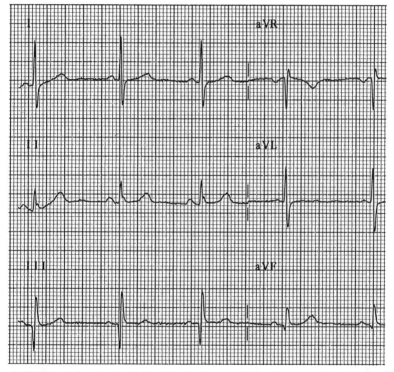

FIGURE 1–2 *Continued*   **D,** Limb leads of a normal ECG showing a deep but normal Q wave in lead III; see Table 1–1 for normal parameters.

Figure continued on following page

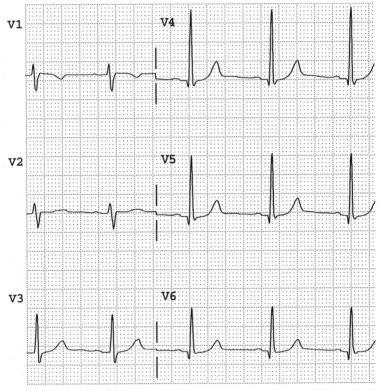

FIGURE 1–2 *Continued*   **E,** Leads V_4 through V_6 show small, normal Q waves < 4 mm deep; leads V_1 through V_3 show normal R wave progression.

STEP 1 **Look at P waves and RR intervals in leads II and V₁.**
Look at leads V₁ and V₂; best for bundle branch block.

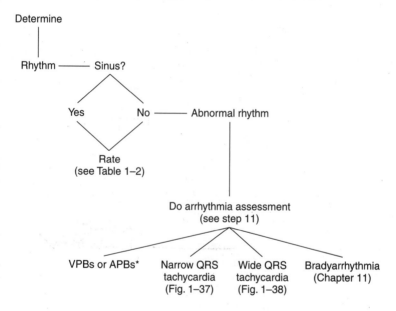

*Ventricular premature beats, atrial premature beats

FIGURE 1–3   Method for rapid ECG interpretation. Step 1: Assess rhythm and rate.

TABLE 1–2   *Determination of Heart Rate*

	HEART RATE (bpm)
NUMBER OF LARGE SQUARES (BOLD BOXES) IN ONE RR INTERVAL*	
1	300
1.5	200
2	150
3	100
4	75
5	60
6	50
7	42
8	38
9	33
10	30
NUMBER OF QRS COMPLEXES IN 6 SECONDS†	
5 × 10	50
6	60
7	70
10	100
15	150
20	200

*Normal paper speed 25 mm/s. One large box or five small squares = 300/min (see Fig. 1–2*B* and *C*).

†If the ECG paper has markers at 3-second intervals, count the number of QRS complexes in two of these 3-second periods and multiply by 10 (see Fig. 1–2*C*). This method is advisable if there is bradycardia or irregular rhythm.

For regular rhythm: start with a complex that lies on a bold vertical grid line.

Rate = 300 bpm ÷ number of large boxes (fifths of a second).

Normal rate between 60 and 100 bpm = 3 to 5 large squares; therefore no need to calculate exact rate.

Or rate = 1500 ÷ number of small (1 mm) squares.

- Do an arrhythmia assessment if the rhythm is abnormal (see Fig. 1–3, step 11 [Fig. 1–37], and Chapter 11 on arrhythmias).
- Determine the heart rate (Table 1–2).

STEP 2: ASSESS INTERVALS AND BLOCKS (Fig. 1–4)

- Determine the PR interval; if it is abnormal (> 0.2 second), consider first-degree atrioventricular (AV) block (Table 1–1).
- Assess the QRS duration for bundle branch block; if it is ≥ 0.12 second, bundle branch block is present; assess both V_1 and V_6. Understanding the genesis of the QRS complex is an essential step and clarifies the ECG manifestations of bundle branch blocks, hypertrophy, and myocardial infarction (MI) (see Fig. 1–5 and Chapters 3 and 4).

RIGHT BUNDLE BRANCH BLOCK (RBBB)

QRS duration ≥ 0.12 second; M-shaped complex in V_1 (see Fig. 1–4); slurred S wave in leads V_5, V_6, and I (see Figs. 1–6 and 1–7 and Chapter 4).

STEP 2

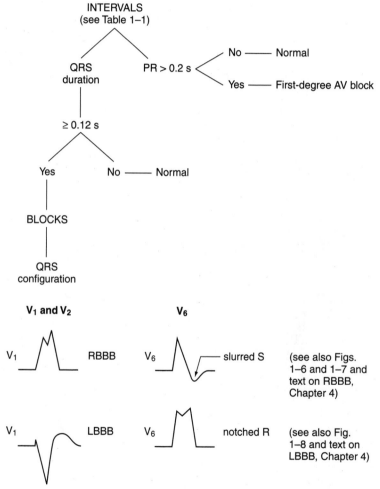

FIGURE 1–4 Method for rapid ECG interpretation. Step 2: Assess intervals and blocks.

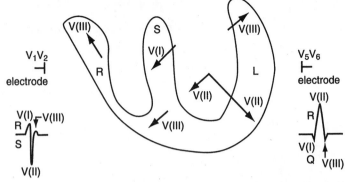

V(I) = vector I produces a small r wave in leads V_1 and V_2, Q in leads V_5 and V_6.
V(II) = vector II produces an S wave in lead V_1 and an R wave in lead V_5 or V_6.
V(III) = vector III produces the terminal S in leads V_5 and V_6 and the terminal r or r′ in V_1, V_2, and aVR.
V_1 = lead V_1 electrode.
V_5 = lead V_5 electrode.
R = right ventricle muscle mass.
L = left ventricle muscle mass.
S = septum.

FIGURE 1–5 Vectors I, II, and III, labelled V(I), V(II), and V(III), underlie the genesis of the normal QRS complex. (From Khan MG. On Call Cardiology. Philadelphia: WB Saunders, 1997, p 51.)

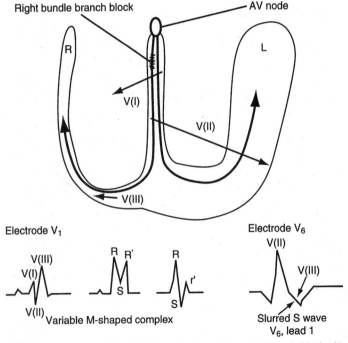

FIGURE 1–6 Genesis of the QRS complex in right bundle branch block. (From Khan MG. On Call Cardiology. Philadelphia: WB Saunders, 1997, p 68.)

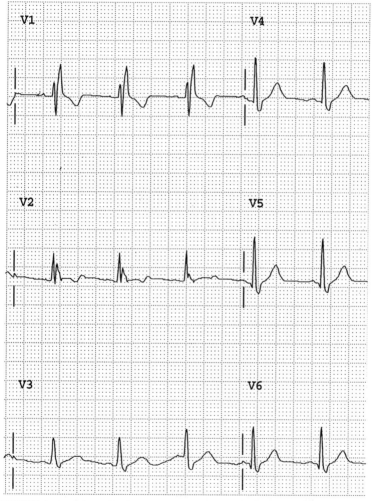

FIGURE 1–7   A, QRS duration in $V_1 \geq 0.12$ second; RSR′ (M-shaped complex) in V_1; wide, slurred S wave in V_5 and V_6: RBBB.   *Figure continued on following page*

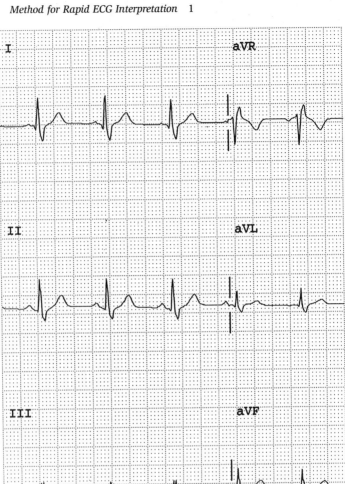

FIGURE 1–7 *Continued*   **B,** Limb leads; slurred, wide S wave in lead I.

LEFT BUNDLE BRANCH BLOCK (LBBB)

QRS duration ≥ 0.12 second; a small R or QS wave in V_1 and V_2; a notched R wave in leads V_5, V_6, and I (see Figs. 1–4 and 1–8 and Chapter 4). In the presence of LBBB, vector forces are deranged and the ECG cannot be used for the diagnosis of ischemia or ventricular hypertrophy. The diagnosis of acute MI in the presence of LBBB is difficult and can be erroneous; see discussion of LBBB and acute MI, Chapter 6.

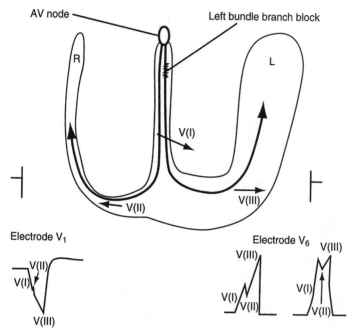

FIGURE 1–8   A, The contribution of vectors I, II, and III, labelled V(I), V(II), and V(III), to the genesis of ~~RBBB~~. (From Khan MG. On Call Cardiology. Philadelphia: WB Saunders, 1997, p 71.)   *Figure continued on following page*

L BBB

2-8

Legend error

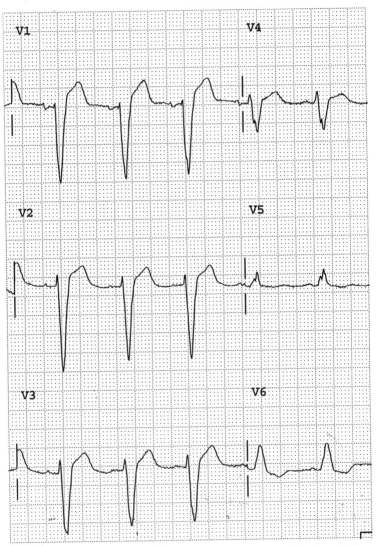

FIGURE 1–8 *Continued*   **B,** QRS duration > 0.12 second; small R waves in V₁ to V₃: notched R wave in V₅; LBBB.

STEP 3 **QRS ≥ 0.11 second but not typical right or left bundle branch block configuration, consider WPW syndrome** (or nonspecific intraventricular conduction delay).

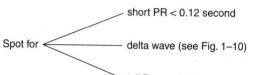

FIGURE 1–9 Method for rapid ECG interpretation. Step 3: Assess for atypical bundle branch block or WPW syndrome (or nonspecific intraventricular conduction delay, Fig. 1–11) (see Chapter 11, WPW syndrome, p. 225).

STEP 3: ASSESS FOR ATYPICAL BUNDLE BRANCH BLOCK OR WPW SYNDROME (Fig. 1–9)

• If the QRS duration is prolonged ≥ 0.11 second and bundle branch block appears to be present but is atypical (Figs. 11–27 and 11–28), consider Wolff-Parkinson-White (WPW) syndrome, particularly if there is a tall R wave in V_1 and V_2 (Table 1–3); assess for a short PR interval < 0.12 second and for a delta wave (Fig. 1–10). WPW syndrome may mimic an inferior MI (see Chapters 6 and 11 for discussion of WPW syndrome). If WPW syndrome, RBBB, or LBBB (Figs. 1–7 and 1–8) is **not** present, interpret as nonspecific intraventricular conduction delay (IVCD) (Fig. 1–11).

STEP 4: ASSESS FOR ST SEGMENT ELEVATION OR DEPRESSION (Fig. 1–12)

• Focus on the ST segment for elevation or depression (Fig. 1–12). ST elevation ≥ 1 mm in at least two limb leads or ≥ 2 mm in at least two precordial leads in a patient with chest pain indicates acute MI, probably Q wave infarction (Fig. 1–13). The diagnosis is strengthened if there is reciprocal depression.

TABLE 1–3 *Causes of Tall R Waves in V_1 and V_2*

1. Thin chest wall or normal variant, early transition (Fig. 1–2C)
2. Right bundle branch block (Fig. 1–7)
   Note: Slurred S wave in leads I, V_5, and V_6
3. Right ventricular hypertrophy (Fig. 7–8)
   No slurred S wave in leads I, V_5, and V_6
4. Wolff-Parkinson-White syndrome (Fig. 1–10)
5. True posterior infarction (Fig. 6–19)
   Note: Associated inferior MI, no slurred S in V_5 and V_6, and T upright in V_1 and V_2
6. Hypertrophic cardiomyopathy
7. Duchenne's muscular dystrophy
8. Low placement of leads V_1 and V_2
9. Dextroposition (Fig. 10–9)

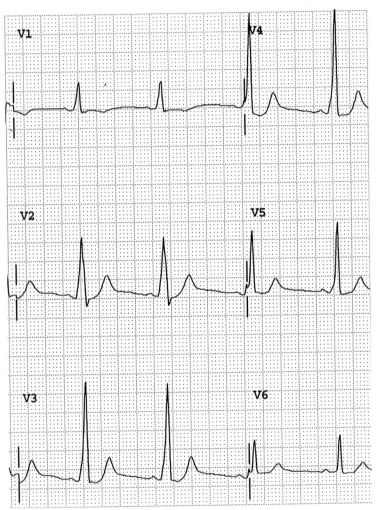

FIGURE 1–10 Tall R waves in leads V_1 and V_2; QRS duration ≥ 0.11 second; delta wave in V_3 through V_5: WPW syndrome.

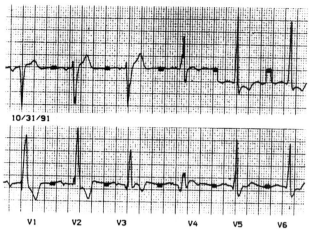

FIGURE 1–11 *Top*, intraventricular conduction delay (IVCD) with normal R wave amplitude in leads V_1 through V_3. *Bottom*, postoperative RBBB with large amplitude R waves in leads V_1 through V_3 stressed a lack of specificity of the tall R waves for RVH in the presence of IVCD, in this instance RBBB. Q waves in leads V_3 and V_4 are consistent with an anterior MI. (From Braunwald, E. Heart Disease: A Textbook of Cardiovascular Medicine, 5th ed. Philadelphia: WB Saunders, 1997, p 147.)

STEP 4

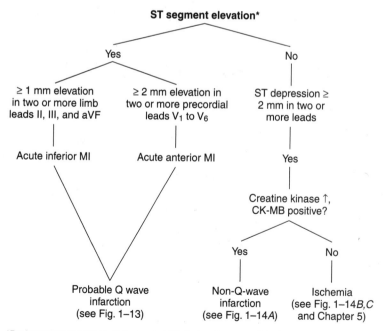

*Reciprocal depression increases probabilities of acute myocardial infarction (MI).

FIGURE 1–12 Method for rapid ECG interpretation. Step 4: Assess for ST segment elevation or depression.

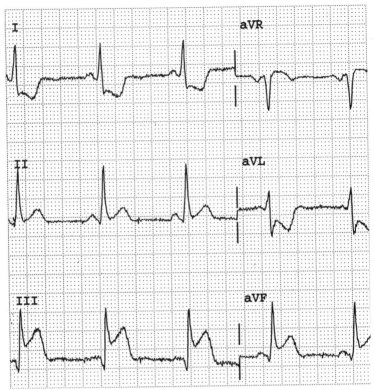

FIGURE 1–13   A, Marked ST segment elevation in leads II, III, and aVF with reciprocal depression in leads I and aVL: acute inferior infarct.

- Figure 1–13 shows features of ST elevation, probable Q wave infarction.
- Figure 1–14A shows features of non-Q-wave MI.
- Figure 1–14B and C illustrates ECG features diagnostic of myocardial ischemia.
- Elevation of the ST segment may occur as a normal variant (Fig. 1–15). See Chapters 5 and 6 for further discussion of ST segment abnormalities and MI.

NOTE: This text advises scrutiny of the ST segment before assessment of T waves, electrical axis, QT interval, and hypertrophy because the diagnosis of acute MI or ischemia is vital and depends on careful assessment of the ST segment.

Exclude other causes of ST elevation:

- Normal variant: 1 to 2 mm ST segment elevation, mainly in leads V_2 through V_4, nonconvex, and with fishhook appearance; common in blacks: even 4 mm ST segment elevation (Fig. 1–15) (see acute MI, Chapters 5 and 6).
- Coronary artery spasm; ST returns to normal with nitroglycerin or with pain relief.

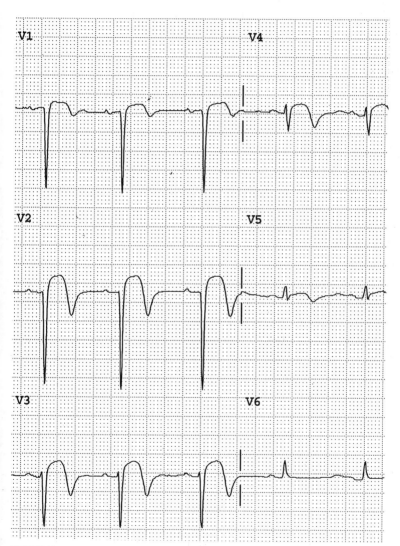

FIGURE 1–13 *Continued* **B,** Marked ST segment elevation in leads V_1 through V_5: acute anterior infarction.

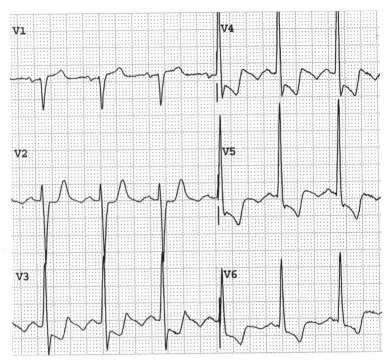

FIGURE 1–14   A, Marked ST segment depression; creatine kinase (CK) and CK-MB elevated: non-Q-wave MI.

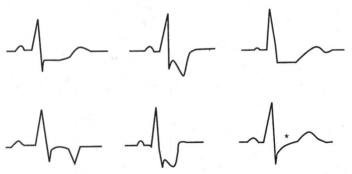

*Upsloping ST depression is nonspecific; commonly seen with tachycardia.

FIGURE 1–14 *Continued*   **B,** ECG patterns of myocardial ischemia. (From Khan MG. On Call Cardiology. Philadelphia: WB Saunders, 1997, p 106.)

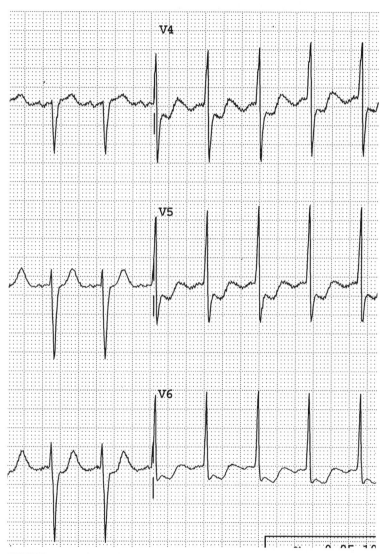

FIGURE 1–14 *Continued*   **C,** Leads V₁ through V₆ show ST segment depression; V₄ through V₆ are in keeping with myocardial ischemia from a patient known to have unstable angina.

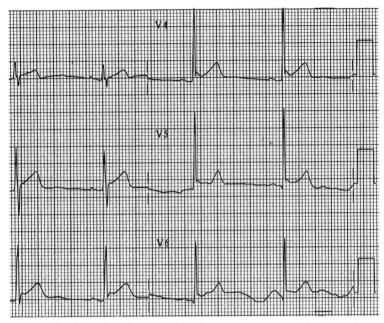

FIGURE 1–15 ST elevation with typical fishhook appearance in the V leads: normal variant.

- LBBB: QRS ≥ 0.12 second and typical configuration (see Fig. 1–8 and Chapter 4).
- LV aneurysm and known old infarct with old Q waves (see Chapter 6).

STEP 5: ASSESS FOR PATHOLOGIC Q WAVES, i.e., LOSS OF R WAVES (Fig. 1–16)

- Assess for the loss of R waves—pathologic Q waves—in leads I, II, III, aVL, and aVF (see Fig. 1–17A,B and Chapter 6).
- Assess for R wave progression in V_2 through V_4. Figure 1–17C illustrates the variation in the normal QRS configuration that occurs with rotation. The R wave amplitude should measure from 1 mm to at least 20 mm in V_3 and V_4 (Table 1–1). Loss of R waves in V_1 through V_4 with ST segment elevation indicates acute anterior MI (Fig. 1–18A).
- Loss of R wave in V_1 through V_3 with the ST segment isoelectric and the T wave inverted may be interpreted as anteroseptal MI age indeterminate, i.e., infarction in the recent or distant past (Fig. 1–18B). Features of old anterior MI are shown in Figure 1–18C and lateral infarction in Figure 1–19.

Poor R wave progression in V_2 through V_4 may be caused by
- Improper lead placement
- Late transition (Fig. 1–20)

Text continued on page 34

STEP 5

a. Assess for Q waves, leads I, II, III, aVF, and aVL.

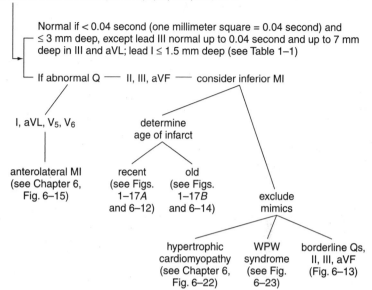

Normal if < 0.04 second (one millimeter square = 0.04 second) and ≤ 3 mm deep, except lead III normal up to 0.04 second and up to 7 mm deep in III and aVL; lead I ≤ 1.5 mm deep (see Table 1–1)

If abnormal Q — II, III, aVF — consider inferior MI

I, aVL, V_5, V_6

determine age of infarct

anterolateral MI (see Chapter 6, Fig. 6–15)

recent (see Figs. 1–17A and 6–12)

old (see Figs. 1–17B and 6–14)

exclude mimics

hypertrophic cardiomyopathy (see Chapter 6, Fig. 6–22)

WPW syndrome (see Fig. 6–23)

borderline Qs, II, III, aVF (Fig. 6–13)

b. Assess for R wave progression in V_1 through V_6 or pathologic Q waves.

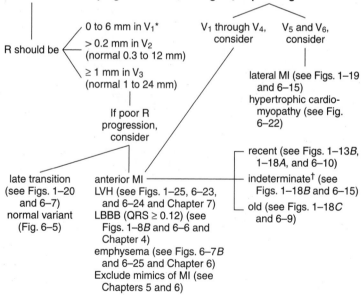

R should be
- 0 to 6 mm in V_1*
- > 0.2 mm in V_2 (normal 0.3 to 12 mm)
- ≥ 1 mm in V_3 (normal 1 to 24 mm)

V_1 through V_4, consider

V_5 and V_6, consider

lateral MI (see Figs. 1–19 and 6–15) hypertrophic cardio-myopathy (see Fig. 6–22)

If poor R progression, consider

late transition (see Figs. 1–20 and 6–7) normal variant (Fig. 6–5)

anterior MI LVH (see Figs. 1–25, 6–23, and 6–24 and Chapter 7) LBBB (QRS ≥ 0.12) (see Figs. 1–8B and 6–6 and Chapter 4) emphysema (see Figs. 6–7B and 6–25 and Chapter 6) Exclude mimics of MI (see Chapters 5 and 6)

recent (see Figs. 1–13B, 1–18A, and 6–10)

indeterminate† (see Figs. 1–18B and 6–15)

old (see Figs. 1–18C and 6–9)

*Age > 30; see Chapter 6 and Table 1–1 for exceptions and normal parameters.
†Compare old ECGs.

FIGURE 1–16 Method for rapid ECG interpretation. Step 5: Assess for pathologic Q waves, i.e., loss of R waves.

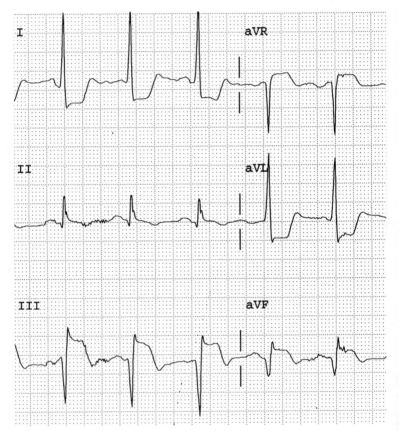

FIGURE 1–17 A, Loss of R wave in leads III and aVF, i.e., pathologic Q waves associated with marked ST segment elevation in leads III and aVF; minimal elevation in lead II and reciprocal depression in leads I and aVL: typical acute Q wave inferior infarct.

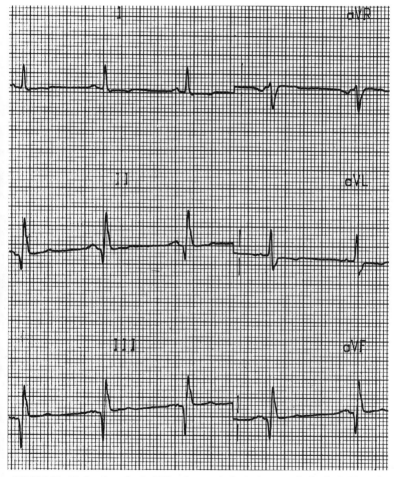

FIGURE 1–17 *Continued*   **B,** Wide, deep pathologic Q waves in leads II, III, and aVF, and the ST segment is isoelectric: old inferior MI.

Figure continued on following page

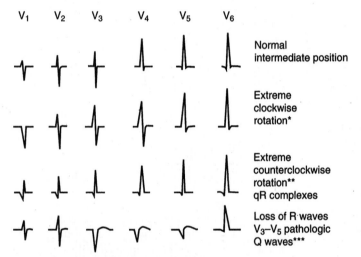

	V$_1$	V$_2$	V$_3$	V$_4$	V$_5$	V$_6$	

Normal intermediate position

Extreme clockwise rotation*

Extreme counterclockwise rotation** qR complexes

Loss of R waves V$_3$–V$_5$ pathologic Q waves***

* = with clockwise rotation, the V$_1$ electrode, like aVR, faces the cavity of the heart and records a QS complex; no initial q in lead V$_6$.

** = qR complexes, q < 0.04 second, < 3 mm deep, therefore not pathologic Q waves.

*** = loss of R wave V$_3$ to V$_5$ pathologic Q waves: signifies anterior myocardial infarction.

FIGURE 1–17 *Continued*   **C,** Variation in QRS configuration caused by rotation. (From Khan MG. On Call Cardiology. Philadelphia: WB Saunders, 1997, p 53.)

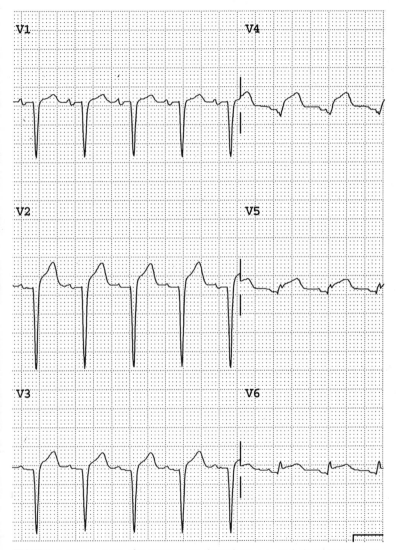

FIGURE 1–18   A, Loss of R waves in V_2 through V_5, i.e., pathologic Q waves associated with abnormal ST segment elevation: acute anterior infarction.

Figure continued on following page

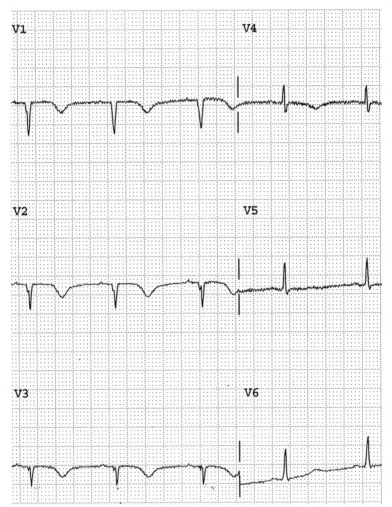

FIGURE 1–18 *Continued* **B,** Loss of R wave in V_1 through V_3, i.e., pathologic Q waves associated with an isoelectric ST segment and T wave inversion: anteroseptal infarction, age indeterminate, infarction occurring approximately 1 to 12 months before the recording of this tracing; comparison with previous ECGs and clinical history required to determine the age of infarction.

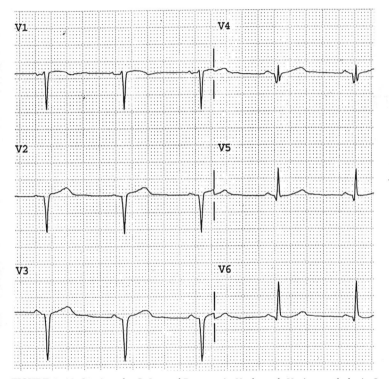

FIGURE 1–18 *Continued*   **C,** Loss of R waves in V₂ through V₅, i.e., pathologic Q waves in V₂ through V₄ not associated with acute ST segment changes: old anterior infarction.   *Figure continued on following page*

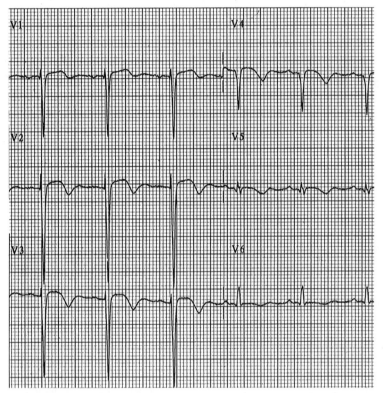

FIGURE 1–18 *Continued* **D,** Loss of R waves in V_4 and V_5: anterior MI, age indeterminate.

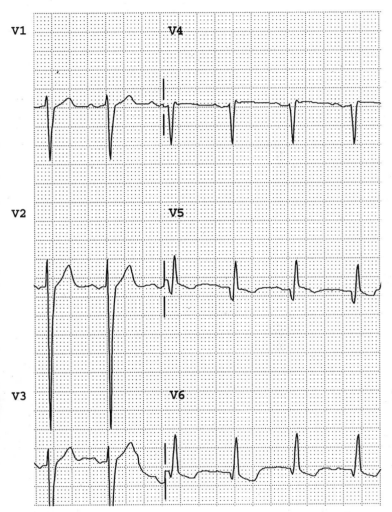

FIGURE 1–19   Pathologic Q waves in V_4 through V_6 and ST segment in keeping with an old anterolateral infarct; clinical correlation necessary to confirm the presence of an old infarct.

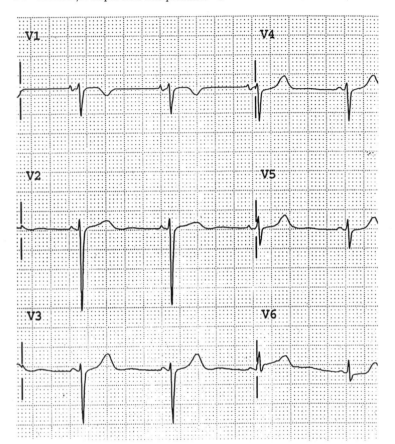

FIGURE 1–20 Poor R wave progression in leads V_2 through V_5; note the negative QRS complex in V_5 is due to late transition and not to other causes of poor R wave progression such as anterior infarction. ECG within normal limits.

- Anteroseptal or anterior MI
- Left ventricular hypertrophy (LVH) (see Chapter 7)
- Severe chronic obstructive pulmonary disease (COPD), particularly emphysema (see Chapter 6)
- Hypertrophic cardiomyopathy
- LBBB (Fig. 1–8*B*)
- In women, albeit rarely, the R wave in V_2 or V_3 may be ≤ 1 mm tall; this may cause an erroneous diagnosis of anteroseptal infarction.

STEP 6: ASSESS P WAVES (Fig. 1–21)

- Assess the P waves for abnormalities including atrial hypertrophy (Figs. 1–22 and 1–23).

STEP 6   Assess P waves in leads II and V₁ for hypertrophy.

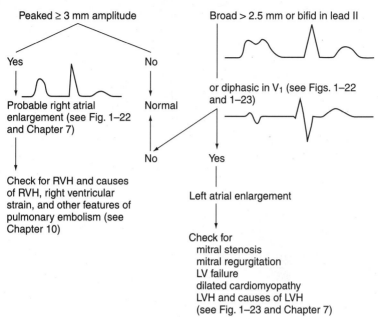

FIGURE 1–21   Method for rapid ECG interpretation. Step 6: Assess P waves.

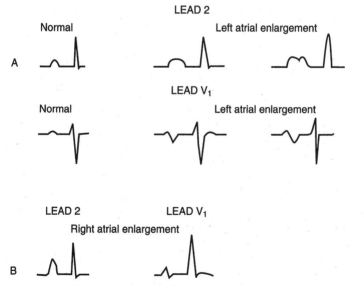

FIGURE 1–22   **A,** Left atrial enlargement: P wave duration ≥ 3 small squares (0.12 second) in lead 2; in lead V₁ the negative component of the P wave occupies at least one small box: 1 mm × 0.04 second = P terminal force > 0.04 mm/s. **B,** Right atrial enlargement: lead 2 shows P amplitude ≥ 3 mm; in V₁ the first half of the P wave is positive and > 1 mm wide (Figs. 1–23, 7–2, and 7–3). (From Khan MG. On Call Cardiology. Philadelphia: WB Saunders, 1997, p 60.)

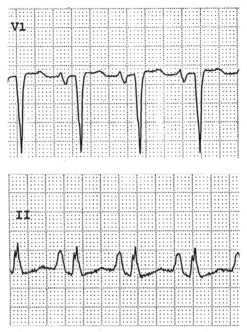

FIGURE 1–23 Lead V_1 shows right and left atrial hypertrophy. Lead II shows peaked P waves caused by right atrial enlargement.

STEP 7

a. **Assess for left ventricular hypertrophy (LVH).***
  (1) S wave in V_1 or V_2 + R wave in V_5 or $V_6 \geq 35$ mm = LVH $\approx 90\%$ specificity; sensitivity $< 30\%$
  (2) R wave in aVL + S wave in men ≥ 24 mm and in women ≥ 18 mm = LVH $\approx 90\%$ specificity; sensitivity $< 40\%$
  (3) Specificity of (1) or (2) increased to $\approx 98\%$ in presence of
    (a) Left atrial enlargement or
    (b) ST segment depression and T wave inversion (strain pattern) in V_5 or V_6 (see Figs. 1–23 and 1–25 and Chapter 7)

b. **Assess for right ventricular hypertrophy (RVH).**
  (1) R wave in V_1 ≥ 7 mm†
  (2) S wave in V_5 or V_6 ≥ 7 mm
  (3) R/S ratio in V_1 ≥ 1
  (4) R/S ratio in V_5 or V_6 ≤ 1
  (5) Right axis deviation $\geq +110°$
    Any two of above = RVH likely (see Fig. 1–26)
  (6) Specificity increased if ST depression and T wave inversion in V_1 to V_3 (see Figs. 1–26, 7–7, and 7–8 and Chapter 7)

*Age > 30; ≥ 40 mm, age 20 to 30.
†Age > 30; see Table 1–1, page 3.

FIGURE 1–24 Method for rapid ECG interpretation. Step 7: Assess for LVH and RVH (not applicable if QRS duration ≥ 0.12 second or in presence of LBBB or RBBB).

STEP 7: ASSESS FOR LEFT AND RIGHT VENTRICULAR HYPERTROPHY (Fig. 1–24)

- Assess for LVH (see Figs. 1–24 and 1–25 and Chapter 7) and right ventricular hypertrophy (RVH) (see Fig. 1–26 and Chapter 7).
- Criteria for LVH and RVH are not applicable if bundle branch block is present. *Thus it is essential to exclude LBBB and RBBB early in the interpretive sequences as delineated earlier in step 2.*

STEP 8: ASSESS T WAVES (Fig. 1–27)

- Assess the pattern of T wave changes (Fig. 1–27). T wave changes are usually nonspecific (Fig. 1–28). T wave inversion associated with

Text continued on page 43

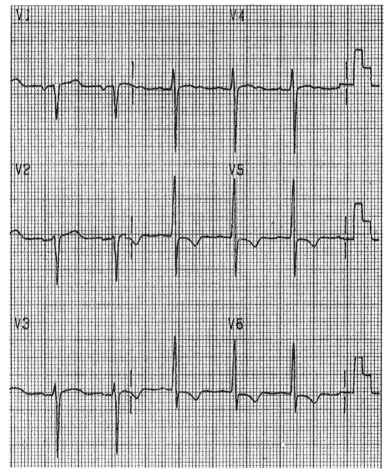

FIGURE 1–25 Note the standardization at half voltage in V_1 through V_6 is markedly increased; ST-T strain pattern in V_5 and V_6; left atrial enlargement; typical features of LVH.

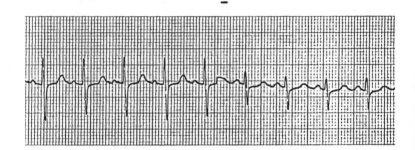

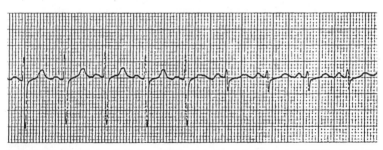

FIGURE 1–26   A, Leads V_1 through V_6: there is a tall R wave in V_1, R/S ratio in V_1 > 1; R/S ratio in V_5 or V_6 < 1: features of RVH.

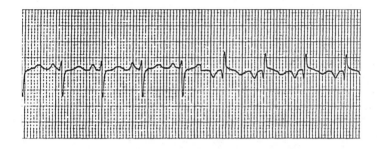

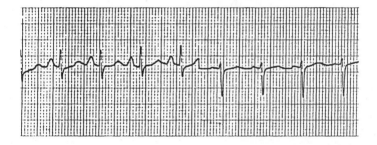

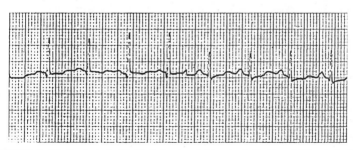

FIGURE 1–26 *Continued* **B,** Limb leads: right axis deviation +140°, peaked P wave in lead II, right atrial enlargement, all in keeping with RVH.

STEP 8

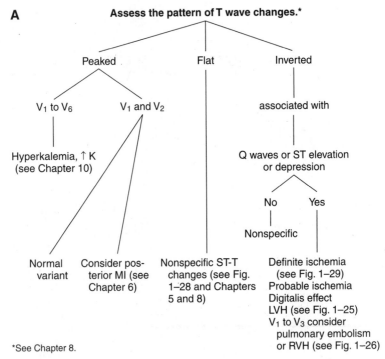

FIGURE 1–27   Method for rapid ECG interpretation. **A,** Step 8: Assess T wave changes.

STEP 8 *Continued*

B **Assess the pattern of T wave changes.**

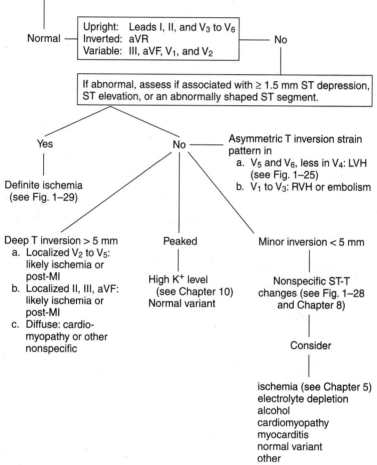

FIGURE 1–27 *Continued* **B,** Step 8: Alternative approach for the assessment of T wave changes.

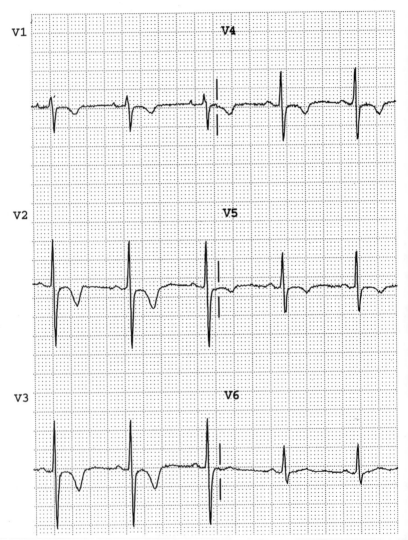

FIGURE 1–28   T wave inversion in V_2 through V_5 not associated with ST segment depression or elevation; nonspecific ST-T wave changes; cannot exclude ischemia, but the tracing is not diagnostic. Abnormal ECG.

ST segment depression or elevation indicates myocardial ischemia (Fig. 1–29). See Chapter 8 for further information on T wave abnormalities.

STEP 9: ASSESS ELECTRICAL AXIS (Fig. 1–30)

Assess the electrical axis (Fig. 1–30). Use two simple clues:
- If leads I and aVF are upright, the axis is normal.
- The axis is perpendicular to the lead with the most equiphasic or smallest QRS deflection (Fig. 1–30*B*). Figure 1–31 shows left axis deviation and the commonly associated left anterior fascicular block (LAFB); see Chapter 9.

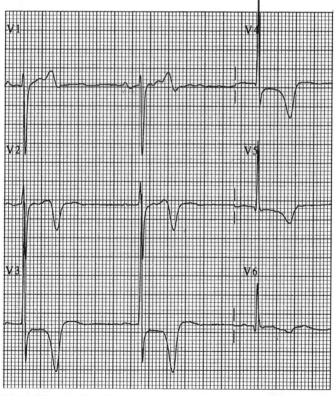

FIGURE 1–29 The deep T wave inversion in V_2 through V_5, which is associated with an abnormal ST segment that is hitched up in V_2 and abnormally coved in V_3 and V_4, is in keeping with myocardial ischemia and likely left anterior descending artery obstruction. Tracing from a 52-year-old woman with unstable angina; tracing taken in the absence of chest pain.

STEP 9

Axis

Rule I

QRS upright leads I and aVF?

Yes

Normal
0° to +110° age < 40
−30° to +90° age > 40

No

QRS positive
in lead I and
negative in aVF

Left
−30° to −90°
(see Fig. 1–30B)

QRS negative
in lead I and
positive in aVF

Right
+110° to +180°

Rule II

Locate the smallest or
most equiphasic lead

Axis is perpendicular to this
lead and in quadrant determined
in rule I above (see Fig. 1–30B)

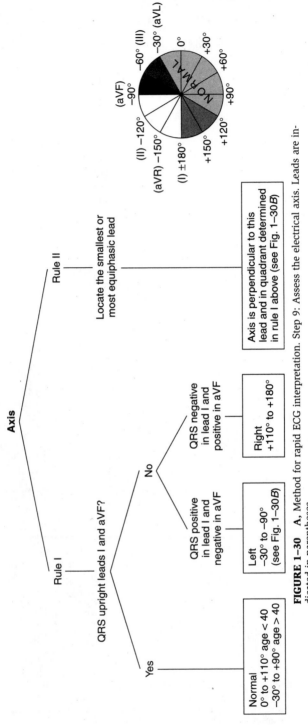

FIGURE 1–30 A, Method for rapid ECG interpretation. Step 9: Assess the electrical axis. Leads are indicated in parentheses.

44

STEP 9   *Continued*

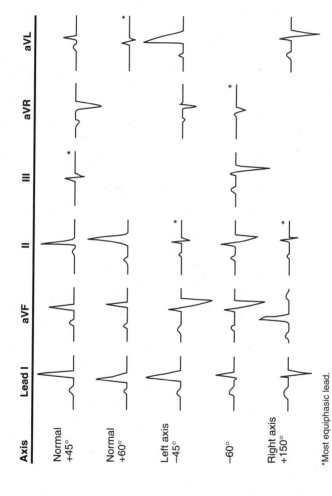

FIGURE 1-30 *Continued*   **B,** See Table 1-4 and Figures 9-4 and 9-5.

*Most equiphasic lead.

TABLE 1–4 *Electrical Axis*

MOST EQUIPHASIC LEAD	LEAD PERPENDICULAR*	AXIS
		Leads I and aVF positive = Normal axis
III	aVR	Normal = +30°
aVL	II	Normal = +60°
		Lead I positive and aVF negative = Left axis
II	aVL (QRS positive)	Left = −30°
aVR	III (QRS negative)	Left = −60°
I	aVF (QRS negative)	Left = −90°
		Lead I negative and aVF positive = Right axis
aVR	III (QRS positive)	Right = +120°
II	aVL (QRS negative)	Right = +150°

*Lead perpendicular (at right angles) to the most equiphasic (isoelectric) lead usually has the tallest R or deepest S wave.

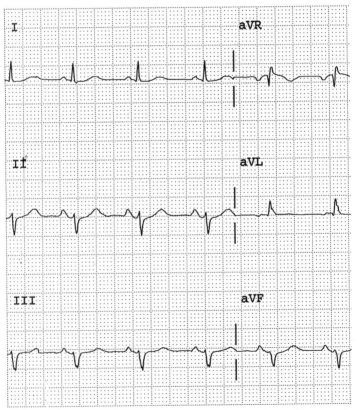

FIGURE 1–31 Lead aVR is the most equiphasic: the lead perpendicular to aVR is lead III, indicating a left axis of −60°. There is a small normal Q wave in lead I and a small R wave in lead III in keeping with left anterior fascicular block (hemiblock). Borderline ECG.

STEP 10: ASSESS FOR MISCELLANEOUS CONDITIONS
(Fig. 1–32)

Do a rapid screen for miscellaneous conditions (Fig. 1–32). Chapter 10 gives details and relevant ECGs.

- Artificial pacemakers; if electronic pacing is confirmed, then no other diagnosis can be made from the ECG (see Chapter 10).
- Prolonged QT syndrome; see normal QT parameters listed in Table 1–5. No complicated formula is required for assessment of the QT intervals (see Chapter 10). Some miscellaneous conditions are illustrated in Figures 1–33 to 1–36.

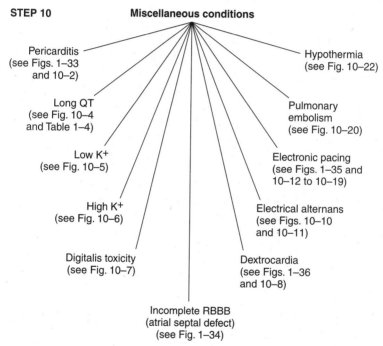

FIGURE 1–32   Method for rapid ECG interpretation. Step 10: Assess for miscellaneous conditions (see Chapter 10).

TABLE 1–5   *QT Intervals* *

HEART RATE (bpm)	CLINICALLY USEFUL APPROXIMATION OF UPPER LIMIT OF QT INTERVAL (second)	
	MALE	FEMALE
45–65	< 0.47	< 0.48
66–100	< 0.41	< 0.43
> 100	< 0.36	< 0.37

*ECG paper speed 25 mm/s. No complicated formula required. See page 174.

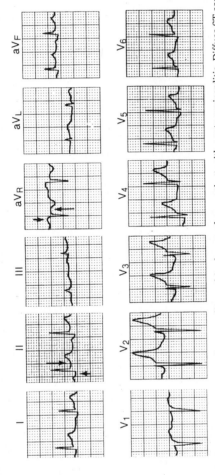

FIGURE 1–33 Stage 1 electrocardiographic changes from patient with acute pericarditis. Diffuse ST segment elevation, which is concave upward, is present in all leads except aVR and V₁. Depression of the PR segment, an electrocardiographic abnormality that is common in patients with acute pericarditis, is not evident because of the short PR interval. (From Braunwald E. Heart Disease: A Textbook of Cardiovascular Medicine, 5th ed. Philadelphia: WB Saunders, 1997, p 1483.)

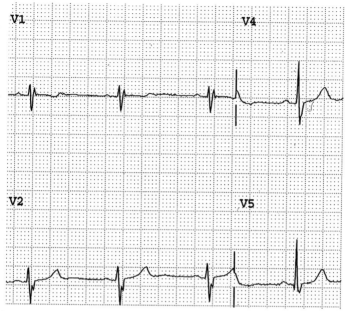

FIGURE 1–34 V leads of a 39-year-old woman who had a large atrial septal defect repaired 5 years earlier. Note the RSr′ in lead V₁ and a wide, slurred S wave in V₅; the QRS duration is 0.1 second: Incomplete RBBB.

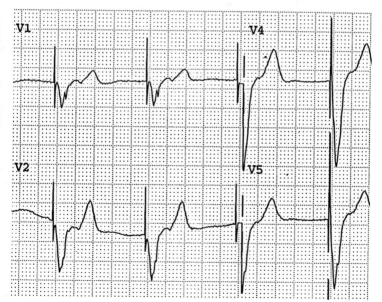

FIGURE 1–35 Shows electronic pacing and ventricular capture; rate = 60 bpm. No further analysis is possible because of pacemaker rhythm.

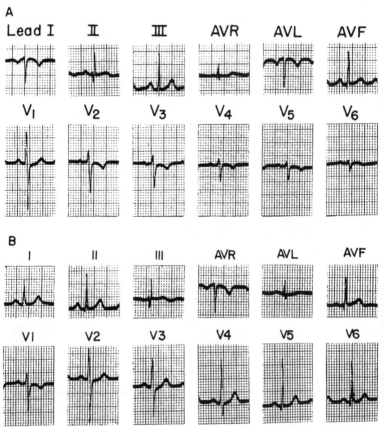

FIGURE 1–36 Mirror-image dextrocardia with situs inversus. The patient is a 15-year-old girl. There is no evidence of organic heart disease. **A,** Tracing recorded with conventional electrode placement. **B,** Tracing obtained with the left and right arm electrodes reversed. The precordial lead electrodes also were located in the respective mirror-image positions on the chest. The tracing is within normal limits. (From Chou TC. Electrocardiography in Clinical Practice, 4th ed. Philadelphia: WB Saunders, 1996, p 313.)

STEP 11

A   **Narrow QRS tachycardia***

Regular	**Irregular**
Sinus tachycardia	Atrial fibrillation
Atrioventricular nodal reentrant tachycardia (AVNRT)	Atrial flutter (with variable AV conduction)
Atrial flutter (with fixed AV conduction)	Atrial tachycardia (variable AV block or Wenckebach)
Atrial tachycardia (paroxysmal and nonparoxysmal)	Multifocal atrial tachycardia
WPW syndrome (orthodromic circus movement tachycardia)	

B   **Wide QRS tachycardia**

Regular	**Irregular**
Ventricular tachycardia	Atrial fibrillation (with bundle branch block or with WPW syndrome [antidromic])
Supraventricular tachycardia (with preexisting or functional bundle branch block)	Atrial flutter (varying AV conduction, with bundle branch block or WPW syndrome [antidromic])
Atrioventricular nodal reentrant tachycardia	Torsades de pointes
WPW syndrome (orthodromic)	
Sinus tachycardia	
Atrial tachycardia	
Atrial flutter with fixed AV conduction	
WPW syndrome (antidromic, preexcited tachycardia)	

*See Chapter 11.

FIGURE 1–37   Method for rapid ECG interpretation. Step 11: Assess arrhythmias: differential diagnosis of narrow QRS tachycardia (**A**) and wide QRS tachycardia (**B**).

STEP 11: ASSESS ARRHYTHMIAS (Fig. 1–37)

Tachyarrhythmias should be analyzed as
- Narrow complex tachycardia. Figure 1–37A gives the differential diagnosis of narrow QRS complex tachycardia.
- Wide complex tachycardia (Fig. 1–37B). See Chapter 11 for relevant ECGs and arrhythmia diagnosis including that of bradyarrhythmias.

ECG TECHNIQUE

- Ensure the standardization is 1 mV displayed as a 10 mm deflection (10 small squares in amplitude).
- Always record the ECG at a standard paper speed of 25 mm/s.
- Remember that artifacts such as baseline drift are often due to loose or improperly installed sensors.
- Most ECG machines have two modes of operation: automatic or manual. Familiarize yourself with the procedure in the ECG department of your own hospital so that you can do the ECG if called at night and there is no technician or nurse available to do the procedure.
- Attach the electrodes (bulb suction cup or flat sensors) on a smooth fleshy part of the upper arm and on the fleshy parts of the lower leg.
- The chest lead sensors are attached as indicated in Figure 1–38 (bulb sensor suction cups or flat sensors).

Ensure that electrodes are properly placed; incorrect lead placement can lead to serious errors with interpretation (Fig. 1–39).

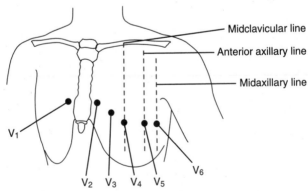

V_1 = 4th interspace at the right margin of the sternum
V_2 = 4th interspace at the left margin of the sternum
V_3 = Midway between positions for V_2 and V_4
V_4 = 5th interspace at junction of left midclavicular line (apex)
V_5 = At horizontal level of position V_4 at left anterior axillary line
V_6 = Same horizontal line as for position V_4 but in the midaxillary line

FIGURE 1–38 Chest leads placement.

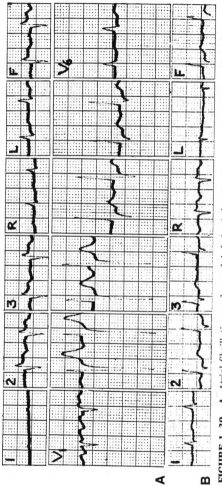

FIGURE 1-39 **A,** Atrial fibrillation and pseudoinferior infarction due to electrode misplacement. With Q waves and ST elevation in leads 2, 3, and aVF and with reciprocal depression of the ST segment in aVL and chest leads, this tracing suggests acute inferior infarction. But lead 1, with virtually no deflections, is the tip-off: The two arm electrodes are on the two legs (and the leg electrodes are on the arms). **B,** Limb leads with the electrodes attached correctly. (From Marriott JLH. Practical Electrocardiography, 8th ed. Baltimore: Williams & Wilkins, 1988, p 469.)

2

The P Wave

The P wave represents the spread of the electrical impulse through both atria (Fig. 1–1). The electrical impulse begins in the sinoatrial (SA) node and depolarizes the right atrium and then the left atrium. Thus the first part of the P wave reflects right atrial activity, and the late portion of the P wave represents electrical potential generated by the left atrium.

FEATURES OF THE NORMAL P WAVE

- The P wave should be upright in leads I and II and in the precordial leads V_3 through V_6 (Figs. 2–1 and 1–2).
- Always inverted in aVR.
- Usually upright in aVF and V_3, but occasionally a diphasic or flat P wave may be seen.
- Variable in leads III, aVL, V_1, and V_2: upright, inverted, or diphasic. (A P or T wave that is partly above the baseline and partly below it is referred to as being *diphasic.*)

FEATURES OF ABNORMAL P WAVES (Fig. 1–22)

- Inverted in II, III, and aVF and upright in aVR: diagnostic of an atrioventricular (AV) junctional (Fig. 2–2) or ectopic atrial rhythm. When there is abnormal propagation of the electrical impulse through the atria, the polarity or axis of the P wave is abnormal.
- Inverted in lead I and upright in aVR, with lead I being the mirror image of I: caused by reversed arm leads or dextrocardia, but in true dextrocardia there is a loss of R wave in V_4 through V_6 (Fig. 1–36).
- Duration ≥ 0.12 second (3 small squares). Most prominent in leads II, III, and aVF; caused by left atrial enlargement (Fig. 1–21). P waves are

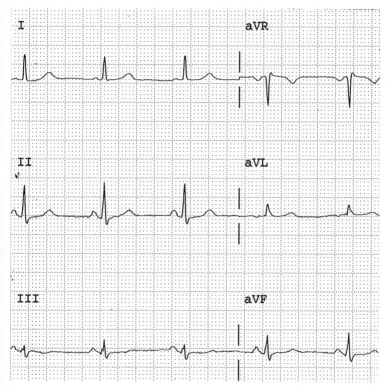

FIGURE 2–1   A, Limb leads of a normal tracing; normal upright P waves are seen in lead I but are best seen in lead II, are inverted in aVR, and usually are variable in aVL and lead III.

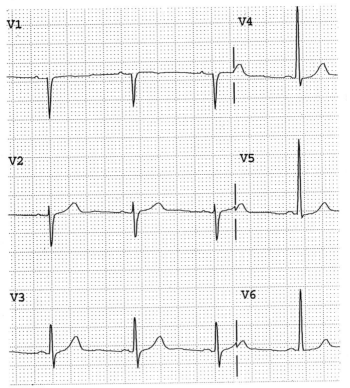

FIGURE 2–1 *Continued* **B,** Same tracing as in *A* showing normal upright P waves in leads V_3 through V_6.

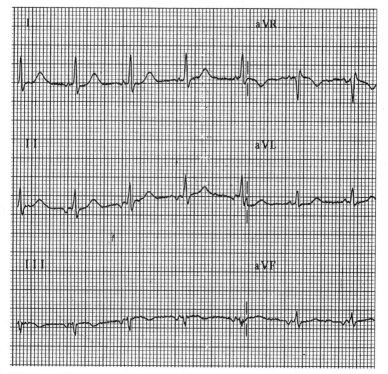

FIGURE 2–2   P wave is inverted in leads II, III, and aVF and is upright in aVR: junctional rhythm.

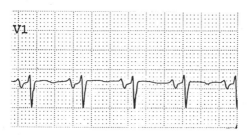

FIGURE 2–3   The second half of the P wave in V_1 is dominantly negative and wide, indicating left atrial enlargement.

seen best in leads II and V_1; thus these leads should be used for rhythm strips and arrhythmia detection.

- Notching of a wide P wave in lead II, III, or aVF: a distance between peaks greater than 0.04 second usually indicates left atrial enlargement (Fig. 1–22).
- Diphasic in V_1: the second half of the P wave is dominantly negative and wide (Figs. 2–3, 1–22, and 1–23). The depth of the inversion times the width represents the P terminal force; if it is ≥ 0.04 mm/s, consider left atrial enlargement, i.e., a negative amplitude of 1 mm with duration of 0.04 second (Figs. 2–3, 1–22, and 1–23). In V_1 the negative deflection is normally < 1 mm.
- Large diphasic in V_1: if the first half of the P wave is positive ≥ 1.5 mm and the second half is negative > 1 mm and wide, consider biatrial enlargement (Fig. 1–23).
- High amplitude, peaking (Figs. 1–22 and 1–23): tall, pointed P waves, taller in lead III than in lead I; high amplitude (> 2.5 mm) particularly in lead II, III, or aVF indicates right atrial enlargement: consider the presence of right ventricular hypertrophy, cor pulmonale, pulmonary hypertension, or pulmonary and tricuspid stenosis. Positive amplitude of the first half of the P wave in V_1 > 1.5 mm indicates right atrial enlargement.
- Absent P waves: consider sinoatrial block and AV junctional rhythms; if the rhythm is irregular, consider atrial fibrillation (see Chapter 11).
- Different morphologies: at least three different P wave morphologies in the same lead: consider multifocal atrial tachycardia (MAT) (see Chapter 11).

3

Genesis of the QRS Complex

Understanding the genesis of the QRS complex is a fundamental step. Knowledge of the normal sequence of activation or depolarization of the ventricles is crucial to an understanding of the normal and abnormal QRS complex. The accurate diagnosis of acute and old myocardial infarction (MI), right and left bundle branch block, hemiblocks, and ventricular hypertrophy depends on knowledge of resultant vectors that dictate the components of the QRS complex.

The electrical impulse that proceeds from the sinoatrial (SA) node activates the atria, producing the P wave, the first wave of the ECG. The electrical impulse is briefly slowed in the atrioventricular (AV) node, then progresses rapidly down the His bundle, the right and left bundle branches, and the Purkinje fibers of the ventricular myocardium. The spread of the electrical impulses through the septum and ventricular muscle is called depolarization and produces the QRS complex of the ECG.

VECTOR FORCES

The electrical impulses that activate each area of heart muscle have direction and magnitude and can be represented by a vector force. The direction of the resultant force can be represented by an arrow, the length of which represents the magnitude of the force. The term *vector* does not imply vectorcardiography.

A vector describes a force in terms of its duration and magnitude. The following three caveats must be considered:

- An electrical impulse travelling toward an electrode causes a positive deflection or R wave (Fig. 3–1).

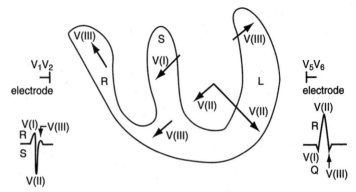

V(I) = vector I produces a small r wave in leads V_1 and V_2, Q in leads V_5 and V_6.
V(II) = vector II produces an S wave in lead V_1 and an R wave in lead V_5 or V_6.
V(III) = vector III produces the terminal S in leads V_5 and V_6 and the terminal r or r' in V_1, V_2, and aVR.
V_1 = lead V_1 electrode.
V_6 = lead V_6 electrode.
R = right ventricle muscle mass.
L = left ventricle muscle mass.
S = septum.

FIGURE 3–1 Genesis of the normal QRS complex. (From Khan MG. On Call Cardiology. Philadelphia: WB Saunders, 1997, p 51.)

- When the impulse is travelling away from the electrode, a negative deflection occurs; i.e., an S, or small Q, or QS wave is recorded.
- Three resultant vectors dictate the inscription of the QRS complex.

Vector I

- The ventricular septum is activated from left to right; an electrode or lead positioned over the right ventricle (V_1) faces the wave of depolarization and inscribes a positive wave, an R wave (Fig. 3–1).
- Because the force of the activation impulse (vector I) is small, the positive deflection is small; the R wave recorded in V_1 and V_2 is small and ranges from 1 to 4 mm in V_1 and from 1 to 7 mm in V_2 in normal individuals over age 30 (see Table 1–2).
- The initial depolarizing current travels away from leads V_5 and V_6 and thus inscribes a small negative deflection, a small Q wave in leads V_5, V_6, and I.

Vector II

- After septal depolarization both ventricular walls are activated simultaneously.
- The impulse depolarizes the thin-walled right ventricle; the magnitude of the forces is small, however, in comparison with the forces that activate the thick left ventricular free wall. Thus the resultant force, vec-

tor II, is directed toward and through the left ventricular free wall (see Fig. 3–1).

- The resultant force, vector II, is indicated by an arrow directed toward the left; the electrodes V_5 and V_6 face the left ventricle and show a positive wave, an R wave, the height of which depends on the thickness of the left ventricular muscle. The height of the R wave in V_4 through V_6 ranges from 10 to 25 mm and may exceed 30 mm in individuals with left ventricular hypertrophy (LVH) and normal subjects under age 25. The R wave in V_4 through V_6 is lost or is reduced to less than 3 mm in height in patients with anterior MI.
- Because the electrical current represented by vector II travels away from an electrode overlying the right ventricle, V_1 and V_2 record a negative deflection, an S wave.
- The larger the left ventricular muscle, the deeper the S wave in V_1 and V_2.

VECTOR III

- Activation of the posterobasal right and left ventricular free walls and the basal right septal mass, including the crista supraventricularis, represents vector III.
- The resultant force is directed to the right and is small in magnitude and may record a small S wave in V_5 and V_6 and a terminal r′ wave in lead V_1 or V_2; thus an RSr′ pattern may occur in normal individuals.

QRS NORMAL VARIANTS AND ABNORMALITIES

CLOCKWISE AND COUNTERCLOCKWISE ROTATION

- Variations in the normal QRS configuration are shown in Figure 3–2. If the heart undergoes strong clockwise or counterclockwise rotation, changes in QRS morphology occur. Failure to recognize these normal variants may result in incorrect interpretation of the ECG.
- With clockwise rotation the V_1 electrode, like aVR, faces the cavity of the ventricle and records a QS complex; therefore Q waves can occur as a normal finding if there is extreme clockwise rotation of the heart (Fig. 3–2). The normal Q wave in V_6 disappears because the resultant force of the initial vector I is not directed toward the electrode V_1.

TALL R WAVES

- If the left ventricle is hypertrophied, the magnitude of vector force II increases; thus a tall R wave is recorded in V_5 and V_6 (Fig. 1–25).
- With right ventricular hypertrophy the magnitude of vector force I increases and tall R waves occur in V_1 and V_2 (Fig. 1–26 and Table 1–3).

Q WAVES

A myocardial infarct is an area of necrotic cells caused by a cutting off of the blood supply to that area of heart muscle. The necrotic area is an electrical window:

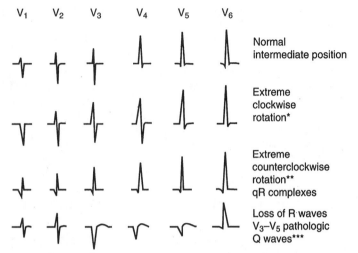

	V₁	V₂	V₃	V₄	V₅	V₆	

Normal intermediate position

Extreme clockwise rotation*

Extreme counterclockwise rotation** qR complexes

Loss of R waves V₃–V₅ pathologic Q waves***

* = with clockwise rotation, the V₁ electrode, like aVR, faces the cavity of the heart and records a QS complex; no initial q in lead V₆.

** = qR complexes: q < 0.04 second, < 3 mm deep; therefore not pathologic Q waves.

*** = loss of R wave in leads V₃ through V₅; pathologic Q waves: signifies anterior myocardial infarction.

FIGURE 3–2   Variations in the normal precordial QRS configuration and correlation with abnormals. (From Khan MG. On Call Cardiology. Philadelphia: WB Saunders, 1997, p 53.)

- If there is necrosis of the left ventricular muscle facing electrodes V₄ through V₆, no R waves, i.e., Q wave, will be produced (Figs. 3–2 and 1–19), or the R in V₃ through V₅ may be considerably decreased; this is termed poor R wave progression (see Chapter 6). Loss of R waves or very poor R wave progression in leads V₃ through V₅ is typical of anterior MI (Fig. 1–18).

- R waves should increase in amplitude from V₂ through V₄. If R waves are present in leads V₁ and V₂ and are not present in V₄ through V₆, consider a diagnosis of anterolateral MI (Fig. 1–19).

- Infarction of the ventricular septum causes the loss of vector I, as well as loss of the normal R wave in leads V₁ and V₂, i.e., pathologic Q waves indicating anteroseptal infarction (Fig. 1–18*A*).

- Normal Q waves are < 0.04 second in duration and are < 3 mm deep. These small Q waves are recorded when a small activation current is directed away from the electrode. Small Q waves are found normally in leads V₅, V₆, and I (Fig. 1–2). Changes in the position of the heart may cause small Q waves in leads III, aVF, and aVL; with extreme counterclockwise rotation small Q waves occur in V₁ through V₆ (Fig. 3–2).

- Leads III and aVL may record narrow Q waves up to 7 mm deep in normal individuals. In lead III the Q wave can be normally ≤ 0.04 second wide and up to 7 mm deep (Fig. 1–2*D*). In all other leads Q waves should be considered normal if < 0.04 second wide and < 3 mm deep.

If Q waves are not observed in lead II or aVF, a Q wave in lead III should be considered normal (see Table 1–1).

- Hypertrophy of the interventricular septum occurs in hypertrophic cardiomyopathy (HCM), and the ECG often reveals deep Q waves that can mimic MI (see Chapter 6).

- When the arm leads are inadvertently placed on the legs and vice versa, Q waves are recorded in leads II, III, and aVF; consider this technical error if there is no deflection in lead I (Fig. 1–39).

- Replacement of ventricular muscle by tumor, fibrosis, or amyloid, sarcoid, or other granuloma may cause an electrical window and Q waves that simulate infarction.

- Lead aVR normally records a negative QRS or QS complex because aVR looks into the cavity of the ventricle and faces the endocardial surface; the activating current flows from endocardium to pericardium (Fig. 1–2).

4

Bundle Branch Block

RIGHT BUNDLE BRANCH BLOCK (RBBB)

DIAGNOSTIC CRITERIA

- Wide QRS ≥ 0.12 second.
- A secondary R wave (R′) in V_1 or V_2, i.e., an rSR′, rsR′, or RSR′ complex that often is **M** shaped. The secondary R wave (R′) is usually taller than the initial R wave (Figs. 4–1, 4–2A, and 1–7A).
- A wide, slurred S wave in leads V_5, V_6, and I (Figs. 4–2 and 1–7).
- The axis may be normal, right or left. If left axis is present, consider left anterior fascicular block (hemiblock) (see Chapter 9).

GENESIS OF THE QRS IN RBBB

The typical **M**-shaped complex in V_1 or V_2 is derived from an alteration of the normal vector forces (Figs. 4–1 and 3–1).

- The initial impulse depolarizes the septum normally from left to right. With RBBB, vector I remains intact; the electrical current travelling toward the electrode V_1 positioned over the right ventricle registers an initial small R wave in leads V_1 and V_2 (Fig. 4–1). Because the right bundle branch does not conduct the electrical impulse, vector II is only directed leftward, activates the left ventricle, and records an S wave in V_1 and V_2. Right ventricular activation occurs later, i.e., unopposed by left ventricular activation; the resultant force, vector III, causes a large R, termed R′ in V_1 or V_2. Thus the rsR′ or rSR′ complex depicts an **M** shape. The deflection R′ is usually greater than the amplitude of the small R produced by vector I septal depolarization.
- The unopposed late depolarization of the right ventricle, which causes the R′ in V_1 or V_2, is recorded as a wide, slurred S wave in leads V_5, V_6,

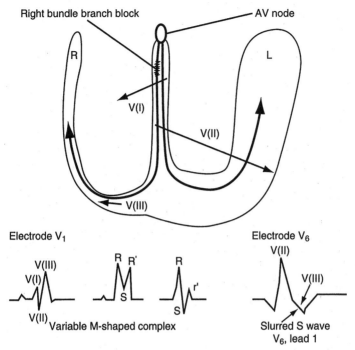

Variable M-shaped complex

Slurred S wave
V₆, lead 1

FIGURE 4–1   Genesis of the QRS complex in right bundle branch block. (From Khan MG. On Call Cardiology. Philadelphia: WB Saunders, 1997, p 68.)

and I, the electrodes overlying the left ventricle (Figs. 4–1, 4–2, and 1–7).

- Because of delayed right ventricular activation, the QRS duration is increased to 0.12 second or more.

CAUSES OF RBBB

- A normal finding in adults at all ages.
- Coronary artery disease and hypertensive and rheumatic heart disease.
- Congenital heart disease, often associated with ventricular septal defect (VSD) and Fallot's tetralogy; with secundum atrial septal defect (ASD), more than 90% of individuals have incomplete RBBB.
- Pericarditis and myocarditis including Chagas' disease.
- Pulmonary embolism and cor pulmonale.
- Cardiomyopathy.

RBBB AND MYOCARDIAL INFARCTION (MI)

- With acute anterior MI, pathologic Q waves occur in V_1, V_2, V_3, or V_4. A Q wave in V_1 and V_2 is not sufficient evidence for the diagnosis of MI.

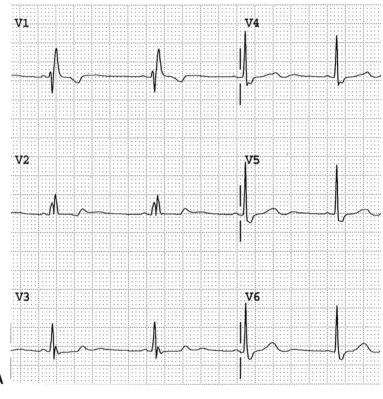

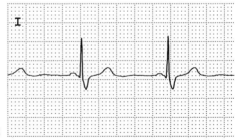

FIGURE 4–2 **A,** An rSR′ in V_1; M-shaped complex in V_1 and V_2; QRS duration ≥ 0.12 second; wide, slurred S wave in V_5 and V_6: RBBB. **B,** Same patient as in *A*. Lead I, wide slurred S wave: RBBB.

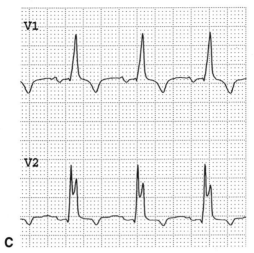

FIGURE 4–2 *Continued*   **C,** RBBB.

- Consider inferior MI only if there are pathologic Q waves in leads II, III, and aVF. Q waves in leads III and aVF are not diagnostic.
- The right bundle branch and the septum are supplied blood by the same artery; thus anteroseptal infarction commonly is associated with RBBB.

Incomplete RBBB

- Incomplete RBBB is a common ECG finding in normal individuals.
- More than 90% of patients with a secundum ASD show incomplete RBBB (Figs. 4–3 and 1–34)
- Confirm the presence of an rSR′, i.e., RBBB pattern, in V_1 or V_2 and an S wave in leads I and V_6.
- The QRS duration should be 0.08 to 0.11 second.

RSr′ Variant

More than 5% of normal individuals show an RSr′ in V_1 or V_2. If the QRS duration is ≥ 0.08 second and there is an S wave in V_5 or V_6 (Fig. 4–3), make the diagnosis of incomplete RBBB. The diagnosis is strengthened if there is a slurred S wave in I, V_5, or V_6.

- If a slurred S wave is absent in lead I, V_5, or V_6 with QRS duration < 0.08 second, the ECG is interpreted as an rSR′, RSR′, or RSr′ variant, borderline ECG (Fig. 4–4); an R′ < 6 mm with an R′/S ratio < 1 suggests normality.

Causes of RSr′ and rSR′ in V₁

- Normal in > 5% of individuals without heart disease.
- Incomplete RBBB.

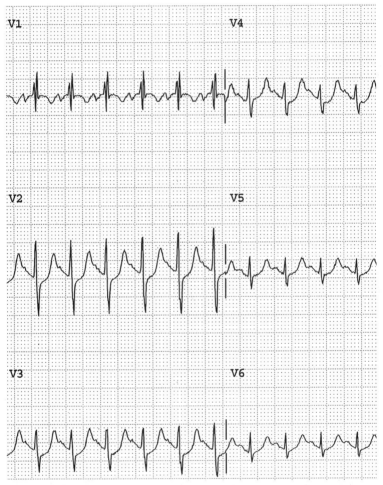

FIGURE 4–3 Sinus tachycardia, rate 147 bpm. QRS duration 0.10 second; rSR′ in V_1: incomplete RBBB.

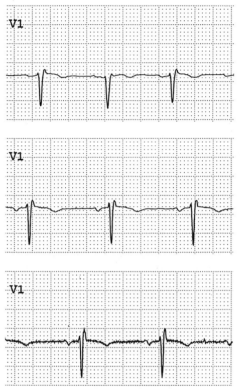

FIGURE 4–4 RSr′ and rSR′ in V₁; recorded in different intercostal spaces.

- Straight back syndrome, pectus excavatum.
- ASD, rarely VSD, and coarctation of the aorta.
- Mitral stenosis and other acquired heart diseases.
- Right ventricular hypertrophy.
- Right ventricular volume overload.
- Cor pulmonale or pulmonary embolism.
- Wolff-Parkinson-White (WPW) syndrome.
- Atrioventricular nodal reentrant tachycardia (AVNRT) (see Chapter 11).
- Muscular dystrophy.
- Late activation of the outflow tract of the right ventricle, the crista supraventricularis, may cause a small, secondary R wave (r′) in V_1.
- Incorrect placement of the V_1 electrode. the RSr′ may appear if V_1 is placed in the third interspace and may disappear with the electrode in the fifth interspace or incomplete RBBB may be recorded (Figs. 4–4 and 1–34). The appearance at a higher intercostal space may be the only abnormality in some patients with a secundum ASD (Fig. 1–34).

LEFT BUNDLE BRANCH BLOCK

DIAGNOSTIC CRITERIA

- QRS duration ≥ 0.12 second.
- A broad monophasic R wave that is often notched or slurred in lead I, V_5, or V_6 (Figs. 4–5 to 4–7 and 1–8*B*).
- Late intrinsicoid deflection in leads I, V_5, and V_6 > 0.05 second.
- Leads V_1 and V_2 reveal QS or rS pattern with poor R wave progression in V_2 and V_3 (Figs. 4–5 to 4–7).
- A presumptive diagnosis of incomplete LBBB may be made if the QRS duration is 0.10 to 0.11 second with notching of the R wave in V_5 or V_6.

GENESIS OF THE QRS COMPLEX IN LBBB

- Depolarization of the left ventricle is delayed, and the QRS duration is prolonged to ≥ 0.12 second.
- The septum and left ventricle are activated by the electrical impulse from the right bundle.
- The normal direction of septal activation from left to right is reversed.
- Vector I flows from right to left through the lower septum rather than left to right. Thus an electrode over the left ventricle records an R wave in V_5, V_6, and I and a QS or rS in V_1 (Figs. 4–5, 4–6, and 1–8*B*).

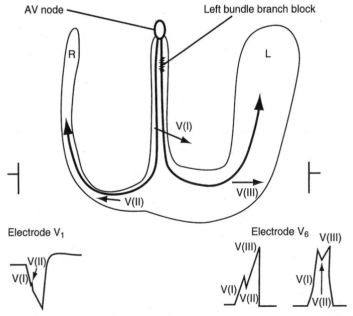

FIGURE 4–5 Genesis of the QRS complex in LBBB. (From Khan MG. On Call Cardiology. Philadelphia: WB Saunders, 1997, p 71.)

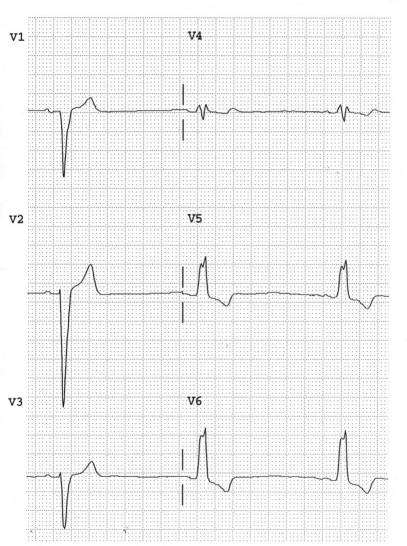

FIGURE 4–6   Sinus bradycardia, 40 bpm; QRS duration > 0.12 second; note the broad, monophasic R wave, notched in V_5 and V_6; poor R wave progression in V_2 and V_3: LBBB.

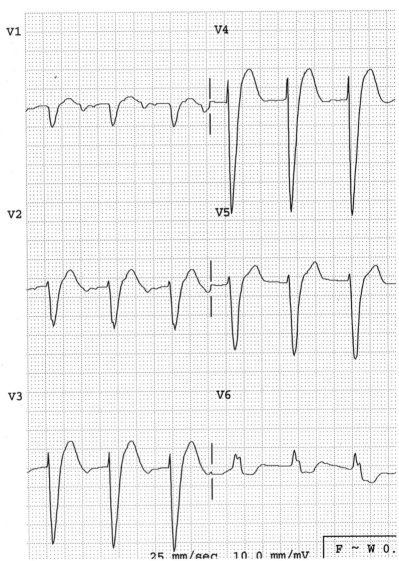

FIGURE 4–7   QRS duration ≥ 0.12 second; poor R wave progression; notched R wave in V_6; note ST segment elevation in V_1 through V_5, typical of LBBB that mimics anterior MI.

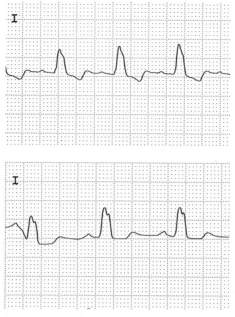

FIGURE 4–8   Notching in lead I: LBBB (two patients).

- Vector II travels from left to right through the right ventricular mass and may cause a slur or notch in the R of leads I, V_5, and V_6 (marked V(II) in Fig. 4–5). The notched R and R′ may result in an M-shaped complex in lead I, V_5, or V_6 (Figs. 4–5 to 4–8).
- Vector III travels right to left and causes and R′ in V_6 (marked V(III) in Fig. 4–5).
- The marked derangement in depolarization of the left ventricle causes the ST segment in leads V_1 through V_4 to be abnormally elevated (Fig. 4–7).
- The ST segment and T waves are opposite in direction to the terminal QRS direction (Figs. 4–5 to 4–7).
- Because LBBB deranges normal vector forces, the diagnosis of left ventricular hypertrophy (LVH) cannot be made in the presence of LBBB. ST elevation, poor R wave progression in V_1 through V_3, and increased voltage are common features of LBBB and do not indicate LVH, myocardial injury, or MI (Figs. 4–6, 4–7, and 1–8B; see Chapter 6).

CAUSES OF LBBB

- LBBB can occur in normal hearts.
- Cardiomyopathies and degenerative diseases.
- Coronary artery disease (CAD); patients with CAD and LBBB have a high incidence of left ventricular (LV) dysfunction and congestive heart failure (CHF).
- Hypertensive heart disease.

5

ST Segment Abnormalities

The ST segment begins after the final deflection of the QRS complex and ends at the ascending limb of the T wave (Fig. 1–1).

Because important cardiac ECG diagnoses are made from observation of abnormalities of the ST segment, the interpreter should rapidly focus on the ST segment; this assessment is step 4 in the method for rapid ECG interpretation (Fig. 5–1). This step is carried out before the assessment for loss of R waves or for the presence of pathologic Q waves, T wave abnormalities, hypertrophy, and axis determination. The diagnosis of acute myocardial infarction (MI), ischemia, and pericarditis depends on careful scrutiny of the ST segment.

Assess the ST segment for
- Elevation: The PR segment is usually used to assess the degree of ST segment elevation or depression. The commencement of the ST segment is usually located at the same horizontal level as the T-P (the isoelectric interval, Fig. 1–1).
- Depression
- Nonspecific changes

Abnormal ST elevation can be caused by
- Acute MI
- Coronary artery spasm
- Acute pericarditis
- Left ventricular aneurysm
- Left bundle branch block (LBBB)
- Left ventricular hypertrophy (LVH)

STEP 4

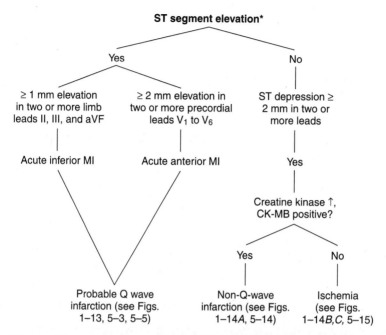

*Reciprocal depression increases probabilities of acute myocardial infarction (MI).

FIGURE 5–1 Method for rapid ECG interpretation. Step 4: Assess for ST segment elevation or depression. Exclude other causes of ST elevation:
- Normal variant 1 to 2 mm ST elevation mainly in leads V_2 through V_4, nonconvex, and with fishhook appearance; common in blacks: even 4 mm ST elevation (Fig. 1–15).
- Coronary artery spasm; ST returns to normal with nitroglycerin or pain relief.
- LBBB: QRS ≥ 0.12 second and typical configuration (see Fig. 1–8*B* and Chapter 4).
- LV aneurysm; known old infarct with old Q waves (see Chapter 6).

ST SEGMENT ELEVATION ACUTE MI

The early diagnosis of acute MI is paramount to the administration of thrombolytic therapy within 15 minutes of the patient's arrival in the emergency room. This early diagnosis depends on the observation of abnormalities of the ST segment and not on the presence of Q waves. Reliance on the presence of pathologic Q waves stems from the proven electrographic principles that were used appropriately from 1930 to the late eighties.
- ST segment depression = ischemia
- ST segment elevation = injury current
- Q waves = necrosis = infarction

With the advent of thrombolytic therapy it became necessary to diagnose acute MI within 1 hour of onset of symptoms, and the diagnosis has to be made without reliance on the presence of abnormal Q waves. Most patients with chest pain and abnormal ST segment elevation in more than

2 leads develop Q waves from 4 to 24 hours after the onset of symptoms. Currently two descriptive terms are used and recognized internationally:

- ST segment elevation acute MI (probable Q wave infarction)
- ST segment depression acute MI (probable non-Q-wave infarction)

The acute injury current of infarction elevates the ST segment and deforms its shape. ST segment elevation patterns of infarction and normal variant are illustrated in Figure 5–2.

Diagnostic criteria for ST segment elevation acute MI (probable Q wave infarct) are as follows:

- Abnormal ST elevation of ≥ 1 mm in two or more limb leads.
- Elevation in leads II, III, and aVF indicates inferior infarction (Figs. 5–3, 5–4, and 1–13*A*). ST elevation in leads I, aVL, V_5, and V_6 indicates anterolateral infarction (Fig. 1–18*A*).
- Abnormal ST elevation of ≥ 2 mm in two or more precordial leads indicates anterior infarction: ST elevation in V_1 through V_3 indicates anteroseptal infarction (Fig. 5–5). ST elevation in V_3 through V_5 (may involve V_2 and V_1) indicates anterior infarction (Figs. 5–6 and 1–13*B*). Extensive anterior infarction is denoted by ST elevation in eight or more leads (Fig. 5–7).
- ST elevation in V_{3R} and V_{4R} associated with inferior infarction indicates added right ventricular infarction (Fig. 5–8). It is advisable to record V_{4R} if the patient with an acute inferior infarct has hemodynamic deterioration.
- Tall R waves in V_1 and V_2 associated with ST elevation in II, III, aVF, or V_{4R} may indicate added posterior infarction. Posterior infarction occurs virtually always in association with inferior or right ventricular infarction. Tall R waves in V_1 and V_2 and T wave upright with no other ECG evidence of MI requires cardiac enzyme confirmation.

Text continued on page 86

A   B

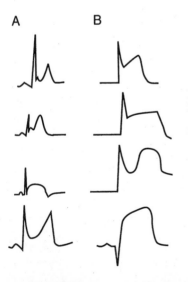

FIGURE 5–2 **A,** ST segment elevation, pattern of normal variant: note "fishhook" appearance; the ST segment usually retains the normal concave shape; the T waves are often prominent and peaked. **B,** Abnormal ST elevation caused by acute myocardial infarction. (From Khan MG. On Call Cardiology. Philadelphia: WB Saunders, 1997, p 90.)

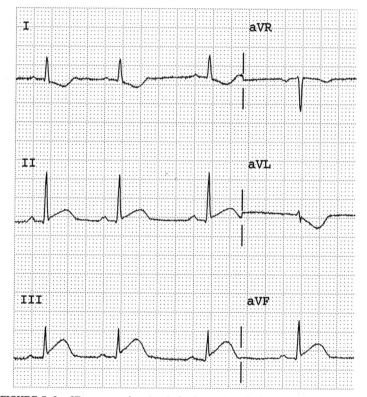

FIGURE 5–3   ST segment elevation in leads II, III, and aVF is diagnostic of acute inferior MI; note reciprocal depression in leads I and aVL strengthens the diagnosis.

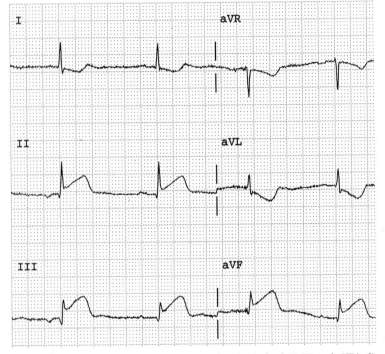

FIGURE 5–4   Marked abnormal ST segment elevation in leads II, III, and aVF is diagnostic of acute inferior infarction; note reciprocal depression in leads I and aVL.

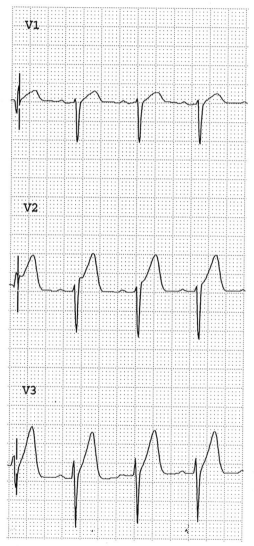

FIGURE 5–5   Abnormal ST segment elevation in V_1 through V_3: consider acute anteroseptal MI. This patient's ECG showed reciprocal depression in leads II, III, and aVF, which strengthens the diagnosis of acute infarction.

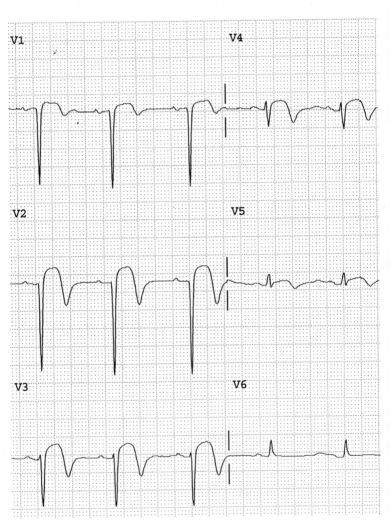

FIGURE 5–6 **A,** ST segment elevation in V_1 through V_5; poor R wave progression in V_2 through V_4 typical of recent anterior infarction.

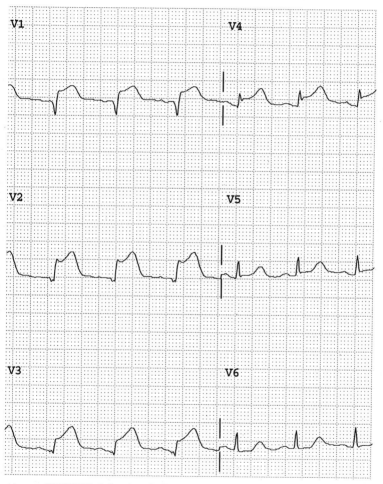

FIGURE 5–6 *Continued* **B,** Variation in shapes of ST elevation.

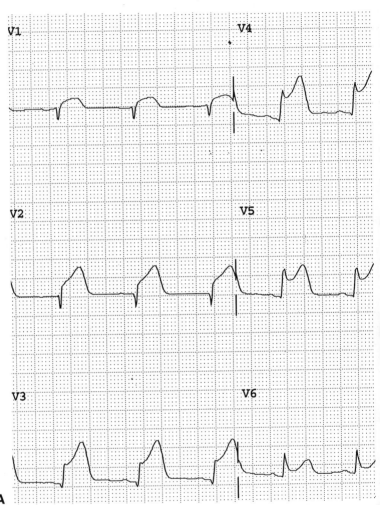

A

FIGURE 5-7   Marked ST segment elevation in eight leads: **A,** V_1 through V_6; **B,** I and aVL: extensive anterior MI. The tracing also showed reciprocal depression in the inferior leads. (From Khan MG. Heart Disease Diagnosis and Therapy. Baltimore: Williams & Wilkins, 1996, p 9.)

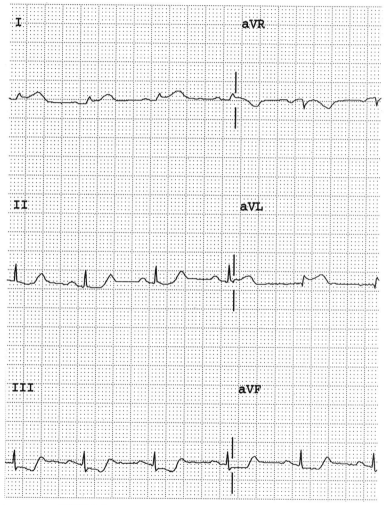

FIGURE 5–7 *Continued* See legend on opposite page.

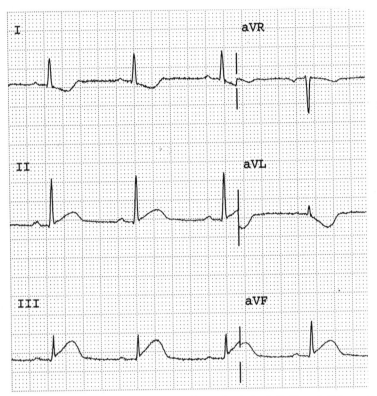

FIGURE 5–8   **A,** Abnormal ST segment depression in leads II, III, and aVF; recent inferior MI.

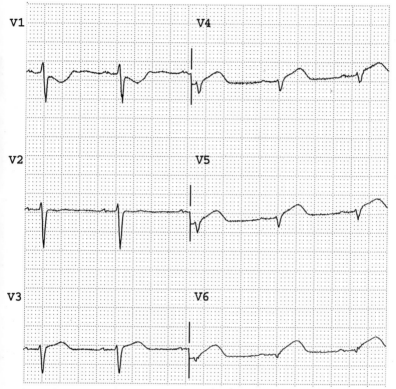

FIGURE 5–8 *Continued*   **B,** Same patient as in *A*. Leads V$_4$ through V$_6$ as labelled are on the right side; leads V$_{4R}$ and V$_{5R}$ show abnormal ST segment elevation. Acute inferior and right ventricular infarction. This tracing was read incorrectly by the computer and cardiologist as "widespread ST elevation, consider pericarditis"; changes in V$_4$ through V$_6$, lateral infarction. (Note V$_1$ through V$_6$ are right sided chest leads.)

Other signs that strongly support the diagnosis of acute MI include the following:

- The simultaneous presence of reciprocal depression is not diagnostic for MI but helps to confirm the diagnosis; this is of particular diagnostic importance because ST elevation that may occur as a normal variant is not associated with reciprocal ST depression. With acute pericarditis, ST depression occurs only in lead aVR and sometimes in V_1 (see Fig. 1–33, Chapter 10, and further discussion in this chapter).
- Evolving Q waves. Q waves become fully developed in 2 to 12 hours from onset of symptoms (Figs. 5–9 and 5–10).
- Diminution of R waves in V_2 through V_4, i.e., poor R wave progression, especially if an R wave is present in V_1 or V_2 and disappears or becomes smaller in V_3 or V_4.
- Evolutionary ST-T wave changes occur during the 10 to 30 hours following the onset of infarction (Fig. 5–10).

An approximation of the size of the infarction can be gauged from the extent of ST elevation:

- Small MI: ST elevation in two or three leads
- Moderate: four or five leads
- Large: six or seven leads
- Extensive: eight or nine leads (Fig. 5–7)

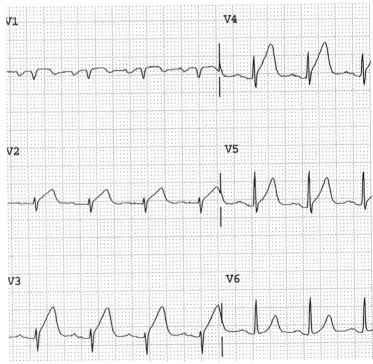

FIGURE 5–9   ST segment elevation in V_1 through V_4; acute anteroseptal infarct.

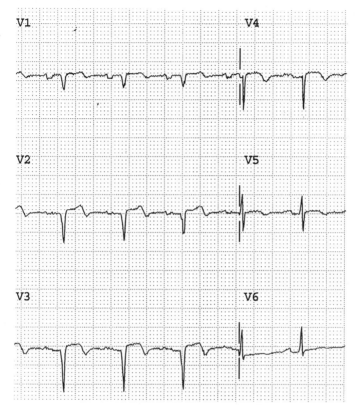

FIGURE 5–10 Same patient as in Figure 5–9. ECG taken 10 hours later shows evolutionary changes; Q waves in V_1 through V_4; convex ST segment elevation is decreased; and T wave inversion has emerged. (From Khan MG. Heart Disease Diagnosis and Therapy. Baltimore: Williams & Wilkins, 1996, p 8.)

MIMICS OF ST ELEVATION INFARCTION

- Normal variants: ST segment elevation is often observed as a normal variant in healthy blacks and some ethnic groups. The ST elevation commonly seen in V_2 through V_5 often shows a notched J point, "fishhook" appearance. This normal variant is inappropriately termed *early repolarization changes.* ST elevation may occur in leads II, III, and aVF, but reciprocal depression does not occur. The degree of ST elevation is variable, often 1 to 4 mm; the normal concave shape remains but may end in a prominent, peaked T wave (Figs. 5–2, 5–11, and 1–15). Occasionally ST elevation with T wave inversion is observed in one or two precordial leads in healthy athletes (Fig. 5–12).

- **Acute pericarditis** causes diffuse ST segment elevation that is not confined to an anatomic coronary blood supply; thus, ST elevation is observed in leads I through III, aVF, and most precordial leads. The ST segment retains a normal concave shape. Reciprocal depression may be

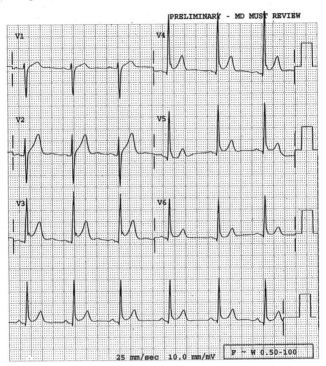

FIGURE 5–11 ST segment elevation in a normal 25-year-old: normal variant; note the notched J-point, "fishhook," appearance in lead V_3. (From Khan MG. On Call Cardiology. Philadelphia: WB Saunders, 1997, p 58.)

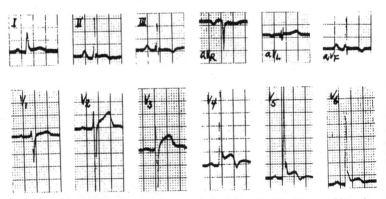

FIGURE 5–12 Benign ST and T wave changes in a healthy 24-year-old professional athlete. The changes, especially in V_4 and V_5, mimic myocardial injury and ischemia and remained the same 15 months later. (From Chou TC. Electrocardiography in Clinical Practice, 4th ed. Philadelphia: WB Saunders, 1996, p 190.)

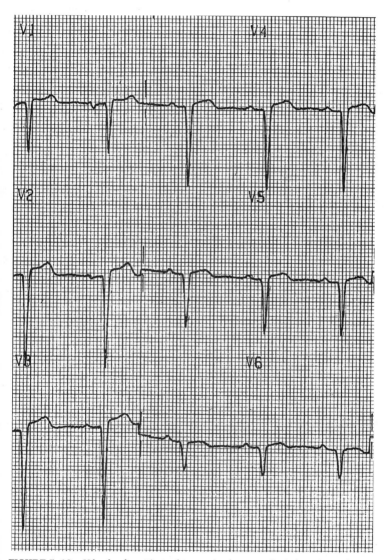

FIGURE 5–13 V leads of a patient who sustained an anterior infarct 6 months earlier: Pathologic Q waves are present from V_1 through V_6, and the ST segment is elevated in V_1 through V_5. The tracing is in keeping with an old anterior MI with left ventricular aneurysm.

observed in aVR and sometimes in V_1 (see Fig. 1–33 and discussion under Pericarditis, Chapter 10).

- **Myocardial infarction age indeterminate** (Fig. 1–18B) in the absence of LV aneurysm may exhibit mild ST elevation, and the differentiation from acute infarction requires clinical correlation and comparison of previous ECGs.
- **Coronary artery spasm,** Prinzmetal's variant angina, causes ST elevation during the brief period of chest pain.
- **LV aneurysm:** ST elevation can persist 3 days to 4 weeks after acute infarction; persistence beyond 4 weeks suggests LV aneurysm (Fig. 5–13).
- **LBBB** nearly always causes abnormal ST elevation in leads V_1 through V_4 and can mimic acute or old infarction (Fig. 4–7).
- **LVH** may cause poor R wave progression in V_1 through V_3, and occasionally ST elevation is observed (Figs. 1–23 and 1–25)
- **Hypertrophic cardiomyopathy** causes Q waves, but occasionally persistent ST segment elevation is present (see Chapter 6).
- **Acute myocarditis** in persons with AIDS may cause nonspecific ST-T changes; ST elevation and Q waves may occur (see Chapter 6).
- **Cocaine** abuse may cause ST elevation and in some frank infarction (see Chapter 6).
- Pulmonary embolism may cause ST elevation (see Chapter 10, Fig. 10–20).

ST SEGMENT DEPRESSION (NON-Q-WAVE) INFARCTION

- ST segment depression ≥ 2 mm in two or more leads in a patient with chest discomfort and an abnormal CK-MB is diagnostic of non-Q-wave infarction (Figs. 5–14 and 1–14A).

ISCHEMIA

ST segment depression indicative of ischemia should fulfill the following criteria:
- > 1 mm depression.
- Present in two or more leads.
- Present in two or more consecutive QRS complexes.
- Flat (horizontal) or down sloping with or without T wave inversion; these patterns of ischemia are all shown in Figures 5–15, 5–16, and 1–14B.
- Abnormal convex coving of the ST segment in V_1 through V_3 or V_2 through V_4 associated with T wave inversion; the terminal portion of the abnormal ST segment has a typical hitched-up pattern (Fig. 5–17); this pattern is often caused by a tight obstruction in the proximal left anterior descending (LAD) artery.

Text continued on page 96

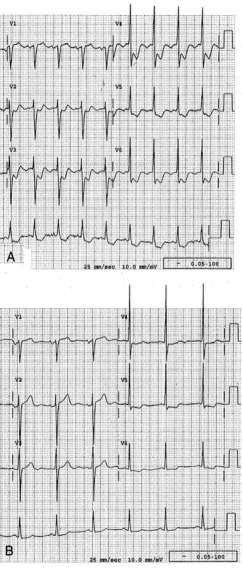

FIGURE 5–14   **A,** Non-Q-wave infarction (acute subendocardial infarction) in a patient with a clinical picture of infarction and elevated CK-MB. Note widespread ST-T depression in the limb and chest leads but no associated Q waves. **B,** The same patient's ECG tracing 18 hours earlier than depicted in *A*. (From Khan MG. On Call Cardiology. Philadelphia: WB Saunders, 1997, p 105.)

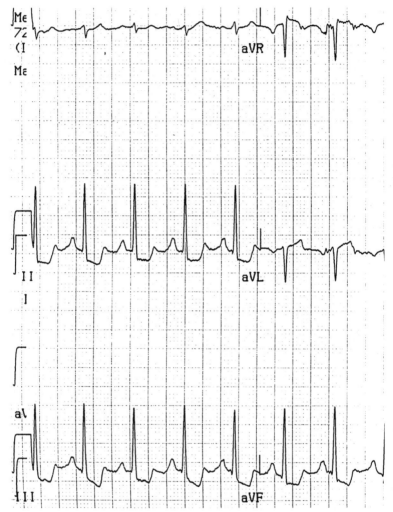

FIGURE 5–15 Flat (horizontal) and downsloping ST segment depression > 1 mm in a patient with proven angina and obstructive coronary artery disease. **A,** Limb leads.

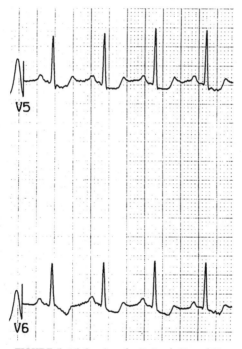

FIGURE 5–15 *Continued*   **B,** Leads V₅ and V₆.

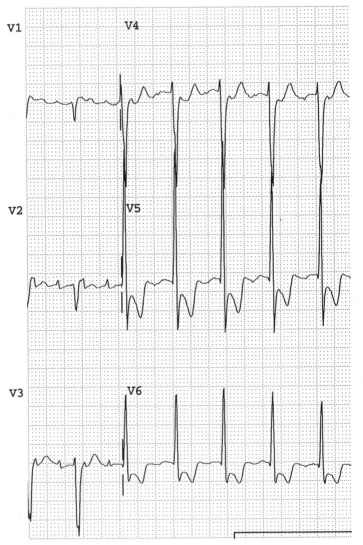

FIGURE 5–16 The V leads of a patient with severe angina and LVH. Note increased voltage and marked ST segment depression in V_4 through V_6.

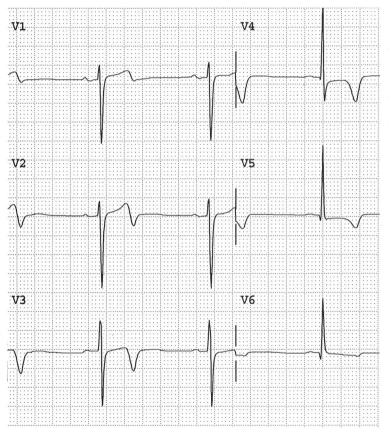

FIGURE 5–17   V leads in a patient with unstable angina. ST-T segment abnormalities seen in V_1 through V_4. The tracing was taken when the patient was pain free. Note the "hitched up" ST segment in V_2 and V_3 with deep T inversion: the pattern is typical of significant proximal LAD stenosis.

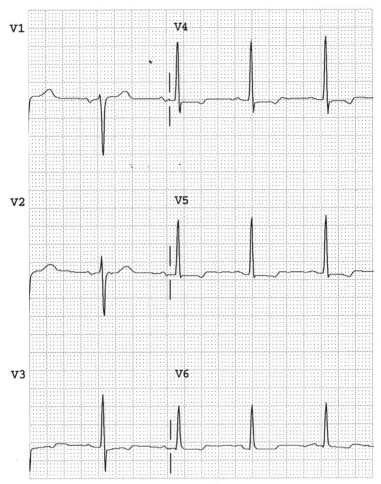

FIGURE 5–18 V leads in a patient with no history of heart disease. ST segment is flat in V_4 through V_6 with minimal T wave inversion; similar finding in leads I and aVL: the anterolateral ST-T wave abnormalities are nonspecific; ischemia cannot be excluded. Borderline ECG.

NONSPECIFIC ST CHANGE

Minor ST segment depression ≤ 1 mm is not an uncommon finding in normal individuals. Consider ST segment changes to be nonspecific if the following prevails:

- ≤ 1 mm ST depression (Fig. 5–18)
- Accompanied by baseline drift
- With or without T wave inversion
- Commonly associated with low, flat, or slightly inverted T waves

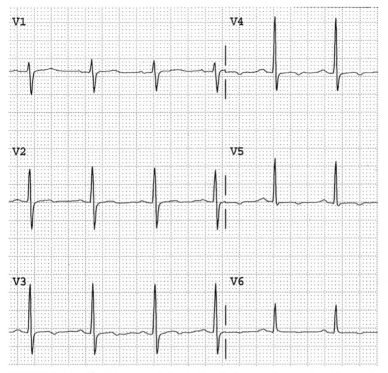

FIGURE 5–19   The ST segment is borderline flat but not depressed and is associated with minimal T wave inversion in leads V_3 through V_6; similar findings were present in leads I and aVL: nonspecific ST-T wave changes. Borderline ECG.

T waves should normally be ≥ 0.5 mm in height in leads I and II. Figure 5–19 depicts nonspecific ST-T changes. Nonspecific ST-T wave changes can be caused by a number of conditions, such as

- Improper electrode contact
- Ischemia
- Electrolyte abnormalities
- Arrhythmias
- Myocarditis
- Pericarditis, constrictive pericarditis
- Intraventricular conduction defects
- Cardiomyopathy
- Pulmonary embolism
- Drink of cold water
- Hyperventilation
- Drug-induced, including ethanol abuse

6

Q Wave Abnormalities

CRITERIA FOR NORMAL AND ABNORMAL Q WAVES

The QRS complex should be assessed for the presence of normal and abnormal Q waves and for normal or abnormal R wave progression as outlined in step 5 of the method for rapid ECG interpretation (Fig. 6–1).

The assessment of pathologic Q or normal q waves should take into account

- Their depth
- Their width
- The leads in which they are observed
- The age of the individual and relevant clinical findings

NORMAL PARAMETERS

- In general a Q wave that is wider than 0.03 second is considered abnormal, except in leads III, aVR, and V_1, in which Q waves may be wide and deep in normal individuals (see Fig. 6–2A and Table 1–1).
- Lead aVR normally records a negative QRS, QS, or Qr complex (Figs. 6–2 and 1–3).
- Normal QS complexes occasionally are found in leads III and V_1 and rarely in V_2.
- A narrow Q wave may occur as a normal finding in lead III; this should be ≤ 0.04 second in duration (1 square) and ≤ 7 mm deep and not accompanied by abnormal Q waves in leads II and aVF (Figs. 6–2 and 1–2D).
- aVL may record a Q wave < 0.04 second and up to 4 mm deep in individuals over age 30 and up to 6 mm deep in children. A negative P

98

STEP 5

a. Assess for Q waves, leads I, II, III, aVF, and aVL.

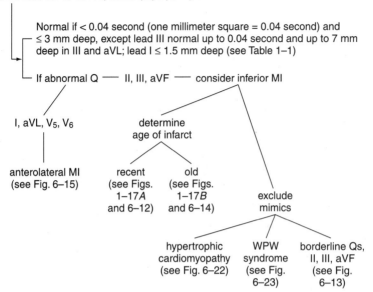

b. Assess for R wave progression in V₁ through V₆ or pathologic Q waves.

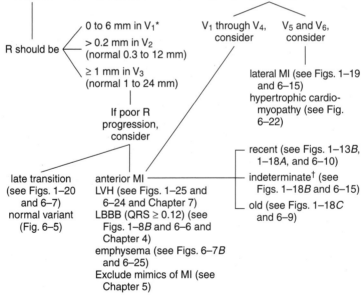

*Age > 30; see text and Table 1–1 for exceptions and normal parameters.
†Compare old ECGs.

FIGURE 6–1 Method for rapid ECG interpretation. Step 5: Assess for Q waves and R wave progression.

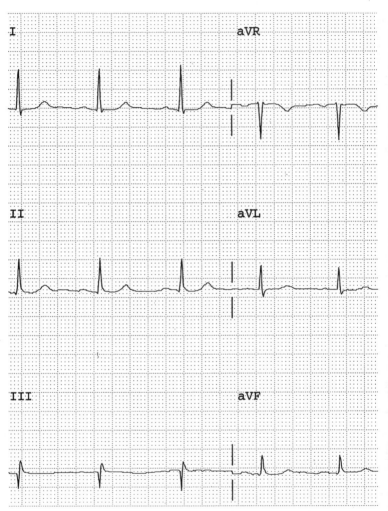

FIGURE 6–2   **A,** Deep, narrow Q wave in lead III is ≤ 0.04 second as part of a normal ECG.

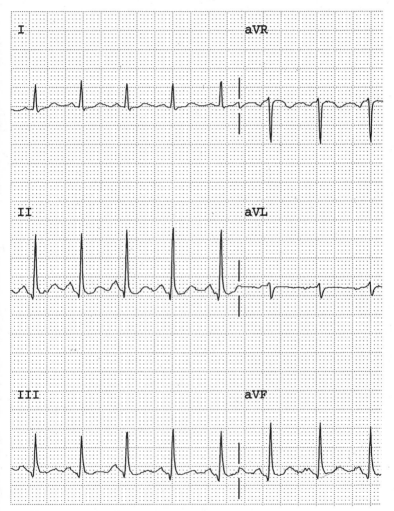

FIGURE 6–2 *Continued* **B,** Note small, normal Q waves < 2 mm deep and < 0.04 second in duration in leads II and aVF. Normal ECG.

wave followed by a QS or Qr deflection with a negative T wave may be recorded in a normal vertical heart.

- In leads II and aVF, small, narrow Q waves may occur but should be ≤ 0.03 second in duration and ≤ 4 mm deep (Fig. 6–2). Occasionally the Q in leads II, III, and aVF are borderline width and the ECG is interpreted: inferior Qs noted; clinical correlation required; borderline ECG.
- In lead I the depth of a Q wave should not exceed 1.5 mm in adults > age 30 (Fig. 6–2*A*).
- In leads V_4 through V_6 and rarely in V_3, normal Q waves ≤ 0.03 second and < 3 mm deep may occur (Fig. 6–3). Normal Q waves should not

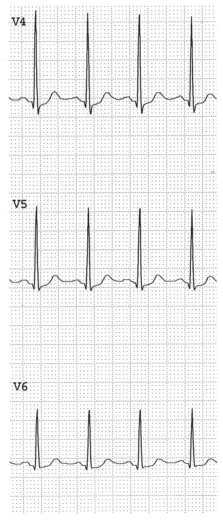

FIGURE 6–3 Normal q wave in V_4 through V_6.

exceed a depth of 2 mm in adults > age 40 (Fig. 6–22) and a depth of 4 mm in those < age 30; rarely an amplitude > 4 mm may be seen in healthy teenagers. Small Q waves may occur in V_2 through V_6 with extreme counterclockwise rotation (Fig. 6–4).

- A Q wave of < 0.03 second and > 2 mm deep in V_2 through V_4 is abnormal if V_1 shows an initial r and there is no marked shift of the transitional zone to the left or right.

- In women and rarely in men under age 30, minute R waves may be present in leads V_1, V_2, and sometimes V_3; this poor R wave progression is not uncommon and may lead to an erroneous diagnosis of anteroseptal infarction (Fig. 6–5).

- Poor R wave progression in V_2 through V_4 with minute R waves may mimic QS complexes and lead to incorrect diagnoses and uncertainties for cardiologists, the attending physician trainee, or family physician. Causes of poor R wave progression include
  – Old anteroseptal and anterior infarction.
  – Left bundle branch block (LBBB) (Fig. 6–6).
  – Left ventricular hypertrophy (LVH).
  – Severe chronic obstructive pulmonary disease (COPD), in particular emphysema.
  – Normal variant in young subjects, particularly in young women (Fig. 6–5).

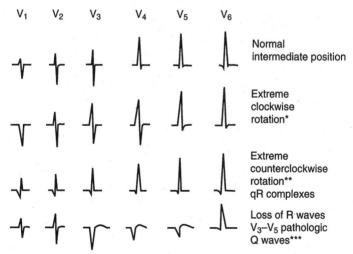

*   = with clockwise rotation, the V_1 electrode, like aVR, faces the cavity of the heart and records a QS complex; no initial q in lead V_6.
**   = qR complexes; q < 0.04 second, < 3 mm deep; therefore not pathologic Q waves.
*** = loss of R wave in V_3 through V_5 (pathologic Q waves): signifies anterior MI.

FIGURE 6–4   Variations in normal QRS configuration and correlation with abnormals. (From Khan MG. On Call Cardiology. Philadelphia: WB Saunders, 1997, p 53.)

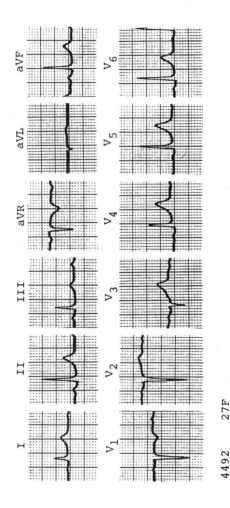

4492   27F

FIGURE 6–5   Poor progression of the R wave from leads V_1 through V_3 in a healthy 27-year-old woman. (From Chou TC. Electrocardiography in Clinical Practice, 4th ed. Philadelphia: WB Saunders, 1996, p 20.)

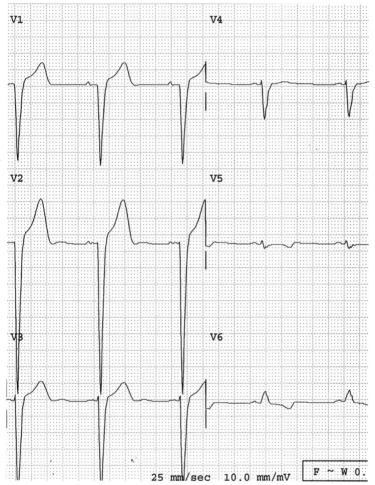

FIGURE 6–6   Poor R wave progression in V₁ through V₄; QRS duration > 0.12 second: LBBB.

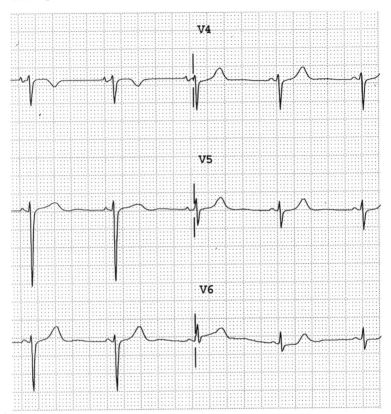

FIGURE 6–7   Poor R wave progression in V_2 through V_4 with normal QRS duration; note that the transition, instead of occurring normally in lead V_3, occurs in V_5 as indicated by a negative QRS in V_5. Tracing from a normal 48-year-old woman: normal ECG.

- – Late transition. A net negative QRS complex in V_5 or V_6 in the absence of right ventricular hypertrophy (RVH) indicates late transition (Fig. 6–7); severe COPD is considered if the P wave amplitude is ≥ 2.5 mm in any of lead II, III, or aVF (Fig. 6–8).
- Note that poor R wave progression in V_2 through V_4 in the absence of late transition, LVH, or COPD suggests a diagnosis of anterior infarction (Fig. 6–9), but clinical correlation is required always.

Q WAVE MYOCARDIAL INFARCTION

Abnormal Q waves caused by myocardial necrosis occur as early as 2 hours and as late as 24 hours after the onset of clinical symptoms of acute MI. Q waves of acute infarction are always associated with abnormal ST elevation.

- The presence of ST segment elevation with Q waves in two or more

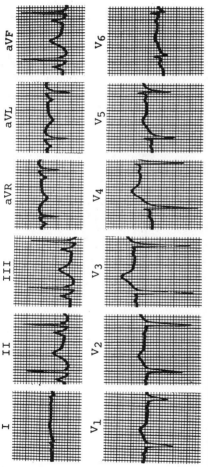

FIGURE 6-8 COPD with pulmonary hypertension. The patient is a 58-year-old man with a pulmonary arterial pressure of 42/25 mm Hg at rest. The ECG shows P pulmonale with a vertical P axis. The QRS complexes in lead I are small, and the frontal plane QRS axis is +90°. There is poor progression of the R wave in the precordial leads, with an R/S ratio in leads V_5 and V_6 of < 1. The amplitude of the QRS complexes in V_6 also is small. (From Chou TC. Electrocardiography in Clinical Practice, 4th ed. Philadelphia: WB Saunders, 1996, p 283.)

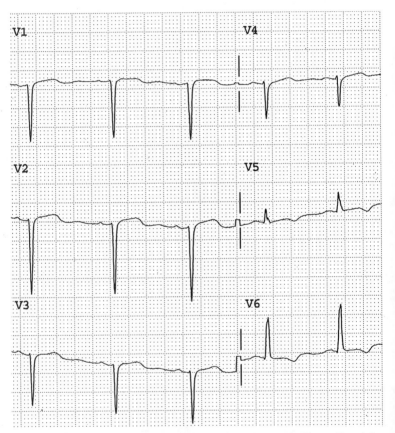

FIGURE 6–9 Poor R wave progression in V_2 through V_4 with abnormality of the ST segment: consider old anteroseptal MI. Note the transition zone is not late in that the QRS complex is not negative in V_5 or V_6; comparison with old ECGs and clinical correlation is required: abnormal ECG.

leads in a patient with acute chest discomfort is diagnostic of acute infarction (Figs. 6–10A,B and 1–13B).

- From 6 to 12 hours after onset of symptoms, ST segment elevation recedes, but Q waves become more prominent (Fig. 6–11).
- Pathologic Q waves in leads II, III, and aVF indicate inferior infarction (Fig. 6–12).
- The Q waves in leads II and aVF should be > 0.03 second in duration, and the Q waves in lead III should be > 0.04 second wide (Fig. 6–12B). An abnormal Q wave in lead III (> 0.04 second in duration) not associated with pathologic Q waves in lead II or aVF should be considered a normal variant. Most of the erroneous diagnoses of infarction are made based on findings in leads III and aVF (Fig. 6–13).
- Pathologic Q waves of infarction may diminish in amplitude and duration during the years following acute infarction. Four to five years after acute MI, pathologic Q waves persist in more than 80% of patients (Fig. 6–14). In some patients abnormal coving of the ST segment and T wave inversion persist for several years and may be difficult to differentiate from a recent infarct; the tracing is often interpreted as infarction, age indeterminate (Figs. 6–15 and 1–18B). In 10%, Q waves become nondiagnostic but still suspicious; in the remaining 10%, Q waves disappear; in about 5% of patients with Q wave infarction the ECG returns to normal. Rarely, infarction may occur in the absence of atherosclerotic coronary artery disease and can be caused by severe coronary artery spasm or cocaine abuse (Fig. 6–16). Also, Kawasaki disease may cause coronary artery aneurysm and MI (Fig. 6–17).

LOCATION OF INFARCTION

- Inferior infarction; pathologic Q waves in leads II, III, and aVF (Figs. 6–12 and 6–14).
- Anteroseptal infarct: QS deflection in leads V_1 through V_3 (Figs. 6–9 and 6–11).
- Anterior infarct: rS in V_1 followed by QS or QR waves in V_2 through V_4 or V_1 through V_5 or V_6 (Figs. 6–10 and 6–11B).
- Anterolateral pathologic Q waves in leads V_4 or V_5 through V_6, I, and aVL (Fig. 6–15).
- Right ventricular infarction is usually associated with inferior infarction. Diagnostic ECG features are ST elevation in V_{4R} and V_{3R} in association with ST elevation and emerging Q waves in leads II, III, and aVF (Fig. 6–18). The ST elevation in V_{4R} recedes within 8 hours of onset of symptoms (Figs. 6–18 and 5–8).
- True posterior infarction occurs virtually always in association with inferior MI. Tall R waves are present in V_1 and V_2 (see Table 1–3). The R/S ratio in V_1 is > 1; the R/S ratio in V_5 should be > 1 to differentiate it from RVH (Figs. 6–19 and 7–7). Q waves should be present in leads II, III, and aVF. Early transition (ET) may mimic posterior MI. In ET there is no pathologic Q wave in leads II, III, and aVF, and the R/S ratio in V_1 should be ≤ 1 (Fig. 6–20).

Text continued on page 127

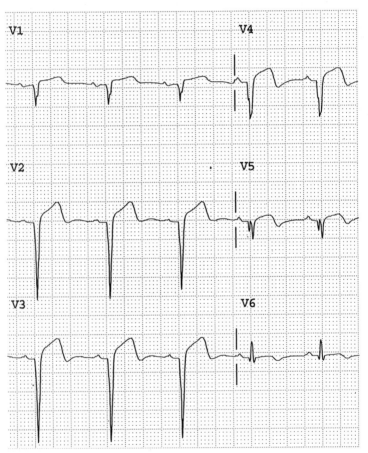

FIGURE 6-10   A, Q waves in leads V_1 and V_2 with marked abnormal ST segment elevation in V_1 through V_4: acute anterior MI.

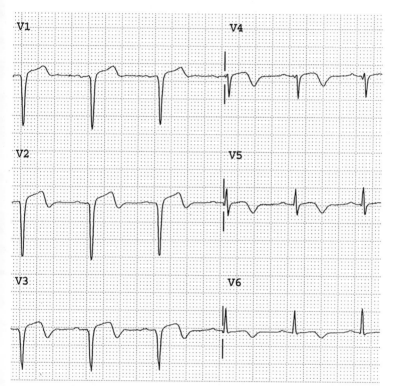

FIGURE 6–10 *Continued*   **B,** Pathologic Q waves in leads V_1 through V_5; abnormal ST segment elevation in V_1 through V_5: large acute anterior MI.

Figure continued on following page

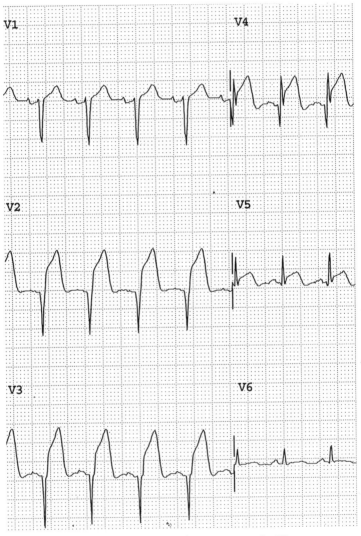

FIGURE 6–10 *Continued* **C,** Acute anterior MI.

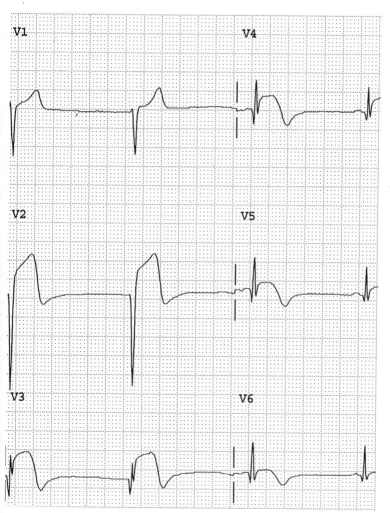

FIGURE 6–10 *Continued*   **D,** Tracing made 1 hour later.

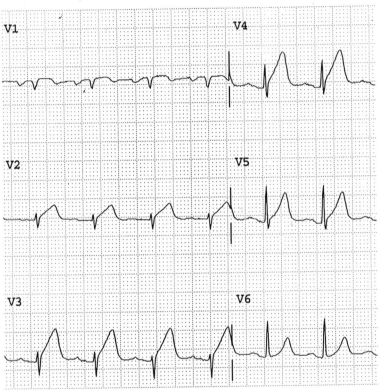

FIGURE 6–11   A, A patient with chest pain and ST elevation in V₁ through V₄: acute anteroseptal MI. (From Khan MG. Heart Disease Diagnosis and Therapy. Baltimore: Williams & Wilkins, 1996, p 8.)

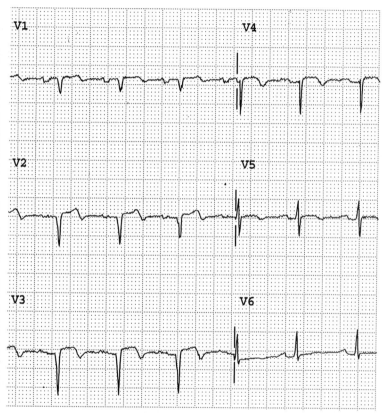

FIGURE 6–11 *Continued*   **B,** Same patient as in *A*. Tracing taken 10 hours later indicates evolutionary changes: Q waves have developed in V_1 through V_4, and T wave inversion has emerged. (From Khan MG. Heart Disease Diagnosis and Therapy. Baltimore: Williams & Wilkins, 1996, p 8.)

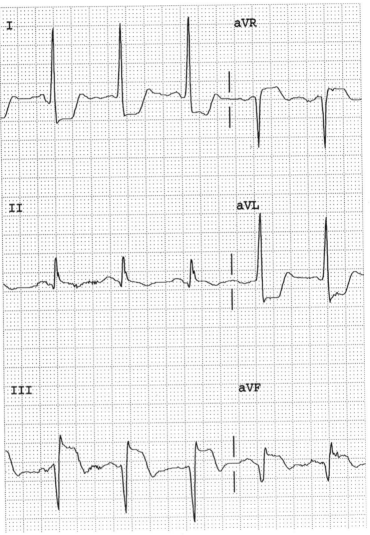

FIGURE 6–12 **A,** Deep pathologic Q waves in II, III, and aVF with marked ST segment elevation: acute inferior MI.

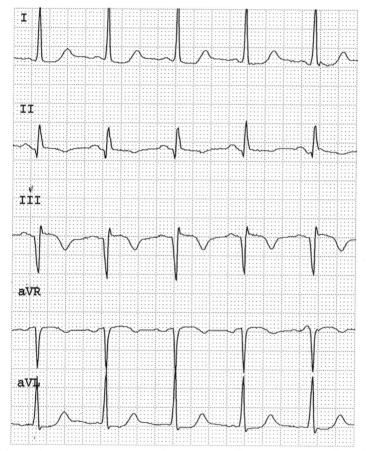

FIGURE 6–12 *Continued*   **B,** Same patient as in *A*. ECG taken 1 hour later shows decrease in ST segment after thrombolytic therapy.

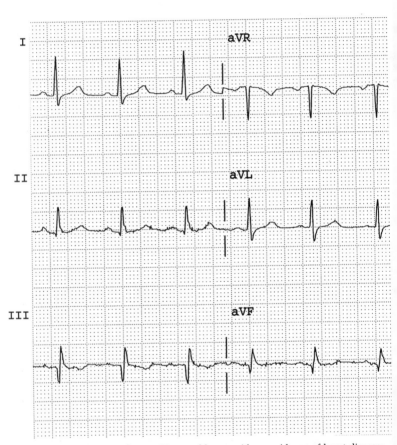

FIGURE 6–13 Tracing from a 49-year-old man with no evidence of heart disease; note narrow small Q waves in leads II, III, and aVF < 0.04 second. Diagnosis: inferior Q waves noted, nondiagnostic, clinical correlation required: borderline ECG.

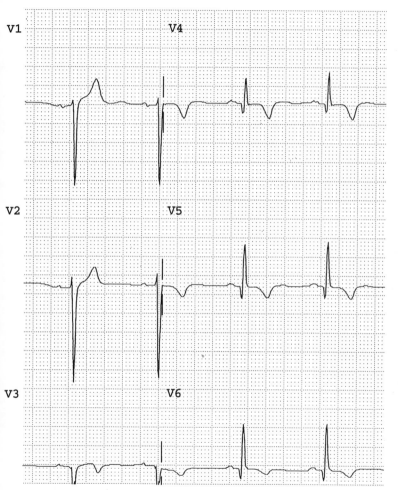

FIGURE 6–14   Pathologic Q waves in leads II, III, and aVF; isoelectric ST segment in patient with old inferior MI.

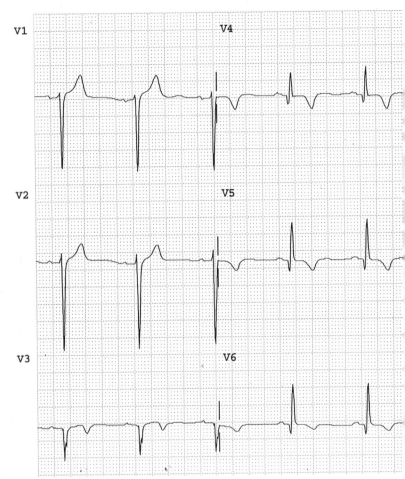

FIGURE 6–15 Another tracing from the same patient in Figure 6–14. Loss of R wave in V_3 through V_6: anterolateral infarct; note the isoelectric ST segment. The ST segment, however, has an abnormal shape with deep T wave inversion, localized to leads I, aVL, and V_3 through V_6: anterolateral infarction age indeterminate. Comparison with old ECGs and clinical correlation required to date the time of infarction.

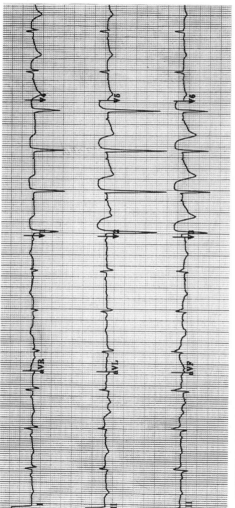

FIGURE 6–16 Acute anteroseptal and inferior MI related to cocaine. The patient is a 30-year-old woman known to be a cocaine user. She developed severe chest pain, and the ECG recorded 90 minutes after the onset of pain revealed ST segment elevation in the anteroseptal and inferior leads (not shown here). Coronary arteriogram revealed complete thrombotic occlusion of the proximal left anterior descending (LAD) artery. Percutaneous transluminal angioplasty was performed with satisfactory result. The visualized artery was long and wrapped around the apex of the heart to supply a substantial part of the inferior wall. The ECG recorded on the next day shows signs of acute anteroseptal and inferior MI. There is a QS deflection in lead V_1, and the R waves in leads V_2 and V_3 are very small. The ST segment in leads V_1 through V_3 is elevated, and the T waves are inverted in all the precordial leads and lead I. In the inferior leads, Q waves are present with ST segment elevation and T wave inversion. (From Chou TC. Electrocardiography in Clinical Practice, 4th ed. Philadelphia: WB Saunders, 1996, p 163.)

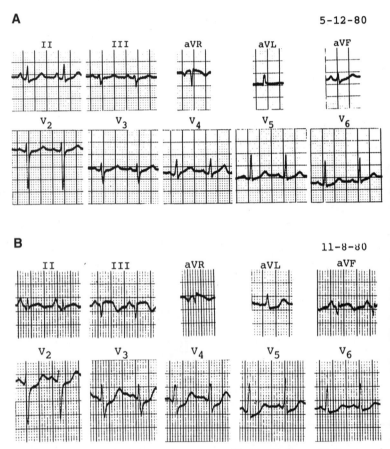

FIGURE 6–17 Acute inferior MI in a 16-year-old girl with Kawasaki disease and coronary artery aneurysm. The aneurysm was demonstrated by coronary arteriogram before the development of MI. The ECG on 5-12-80 **(A)** was obtained before and that on 11-8-80 **(B)** after the infarction occurred. Note the appearance of Q waves with ST segment elevation and T wave inversion in the inferior leads on the tracing of 11-8-80. (Courtesy Dr. Samuel Kaplan. From Chou TC. Electrocardiography in Clinical Practice, 4th ed. Philadelphia: WB Saunders, 1996, p 165.)

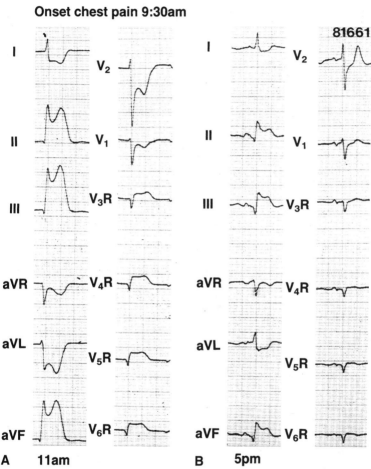

FIGURE 6–18   **A,** Serial tracings from a patient with acute inferoposterior and right ventricular infarction. **B,** Note that the diagnostic changes of right ventricular infarction seen in lead V_{4R} have disappeared $7\frac{1}{2}$ hours after the onset of pain. (From Wellens JJH. The ECG in Emergency Decision Making. Philadelphia: WB Saunders, 1992, p 9.)

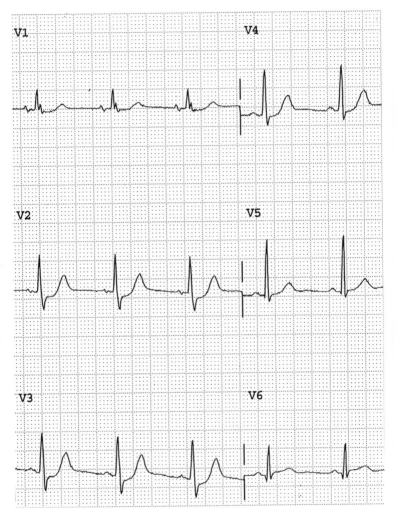

FIGURE 6–19 Note tall R waves in V_1 and V_2 in the absence of RVH, WPW syndrome, or RBBB and thus in keeping with posterior infarction; note upright T wave in V_1 and V_2; limb leads showed inferior MI. (From Khan MG. Heart Disease Diagnosis and Therapy. Baltimore: Williams & Wilkins, 1996, p 11.)

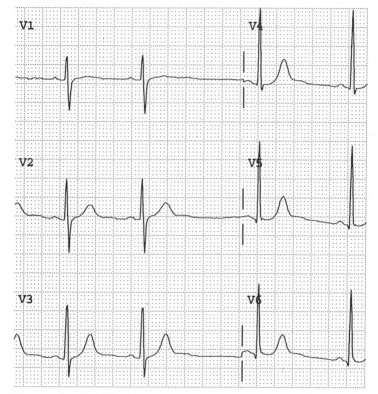

FIGURE 6–20   The V leads in a normal 26-year-old woman. Note the R wave is tall in V_1; QRS is positive in V_2, indicating early transition; there is no posterior infarction; R/S ratio in V_1 is ≤ 1; the limb leads showed no pathologic Q waves in II, III, and aVF, and there is no indication of inferior or right ventricular infarction: normal ECG.

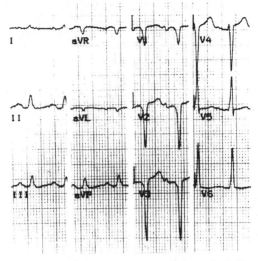

FIGURE 6-21 AIDS myocarditis simulating an anteroseptal MI. (From Braunwald E. Heart Disease: A Textbook of Cardiovascular Medicine, 5th ed. Philadelphia: WB Saunders, 1997, p 149.)

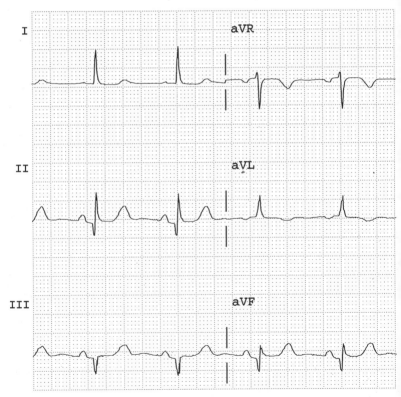

FIGURE 6-22 **A,** Deep, wide pathologic Q waves in leads II, III, and aVF in a 52-year-old woman with known hypertrophic cardiomyopathy.

MIMICS OF Q WAVE MYOCARDIAL INFARCTION

- Myocarditis including Chagas' disease and AIDS (Fig. 6–21) may cause pathologic Q waves.
- Pathologic Q waves may occur in patients with hypertrophic cardiomyopathy (Fig. 6–22).
- Pseudo-Q waves in leads II, III, and aVF in Wolff-Parkinson-White (WPW) syndrome may mimic inferior MI (Fig. 6–23).
- In LVH, QS may occur in lead V_1, V_2, or V_3 and simulate MI (Fig. 6–24).
- Typically in LBBB R waves are absent or minute in V_1 through V_3. LBBB can simulate anteroseptal infarction (Figs. 1–8*B* and 6–6); also Q waves may occur in leads II, III, and aVF in the absence of infarction.
- In some patients with emphysema a QS pattern may be recorded in leads V_1 through V_4 and mimic anterior MI. The precordial leads should be placed one intercostal space lower than usual (Fig. 6–25).
- A left sided pneumothorax may cause a QS pattern in leads V_1 through V_4.
- Massive pulmonary embolism may cause a QS pattern in leads V_1 through V_4 (see Chapter 10).
- Nonpenetration chest trauma may cause Q waves simulating MI.

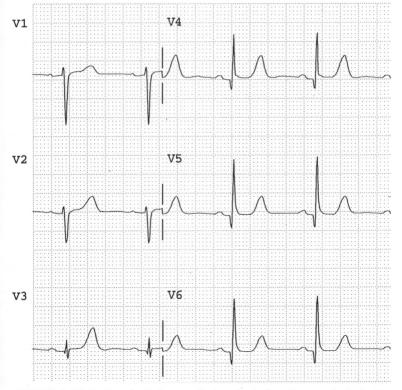

FIGURE 6–22 *Continued*   **B**, Same patient as in *A*; deep Q waves in leads V_4 through V_6.

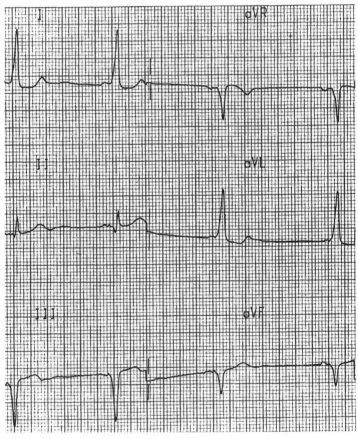

FIGURE 6–23 Tracing from a 42-year-old woman with WPW syndrome; note pseudo-Q waves in leads II, III, and aVF, which can mimic inferior MI.

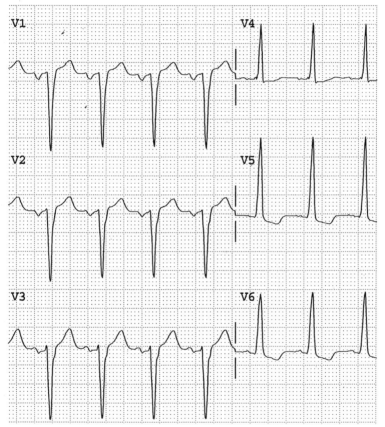

FIGURE 6–24 LVH: QS complexes in V_1 and V_2; a minute R wave in V_3; the tracing can mimic old anteroseptal MI, a common error of interpretation.

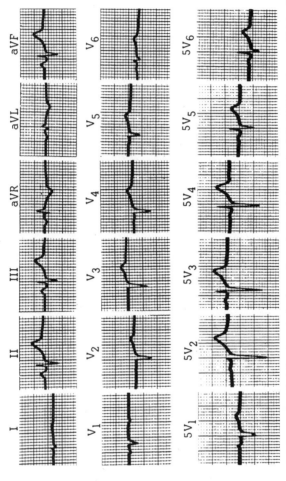

FIGURE 6–25 QS deflections in leads V_1 through V_4 mimic anterior MI. Additional precordial leads were recorded one intercostal space below the levels of the routine electrode locations. ECG of a 58-year-old man with severe emphysema. The QRS complexes are partially normalized. (From Chou TC. Pseudoinfarction. Cardiovasc Clin 1973;5[3]:199.)

LBBB AND INFARCTION

The diagnosis of MI in the presence of LBBB is fraught with possible diagnostic errors, and in most cases a diagnosis of acute or old infarction cannot be made with confidence. The usual finding in LBBB is a QS pattern in V_1 and V_3 or very small r waves in V_1 through V_3 simulating infarction or LVH.

ECG FEATURES SUGGESTIVE OF LBBB WITH INFARCTION

- Q waves in leads I, aVL, V_5, and V_6 indicate an anterior (anterolateral or anteroseptal) infarct (Figs. 6–26 and 6–27), but a false-positive diagnosis is common. These findings often occur in the absence of infarction and may occur in patients with severe LVH or nonspecific fibrosis.
- A reversal of R wave progression in the right and midprecordial leads. R waves in V_1 and V_2 that decrease in amplitude in V_3 and V_4 may indicate anterior infarction, but false-positive diagnoses are common.

RBBB AND INFARCTION

RBBB may be associated with deep Q waves in leads III and aVF without infarction. MI is likely only if there is an added Q wave in lead II.
- RBBB can be associated with Q waves in leads V_1 and V_2 without infarction. Added Q waves in V_3 and beyond suggest infarction.

LOW-VOLTAGE QRS

ECGs should be recorded with the graph paper moving at 25 mm/s. At this speed a 1 mm square on the horizontal plane equals 0.04 second. The voltage of the P wave, QRS complex, and T wave are measured vertically with reference to the calibration or standardization that should be set at 1 mV = 10 mm. With this universal standardization, a 1 mm square in a vertical direction measures 0.1 mV.

CRITERIA FOR LOW-VOLTAGE QRS

- In all limb leads the amplitude of the entire QRS complex (R + S) is < 5 mm.
- In each of the precordial leads the amplitude of the entire QRS complex (R + S) is < 10 mm.

CAUSES OF LOW-VOLTAGE QRS

- Obesity
- Pericardial effusion

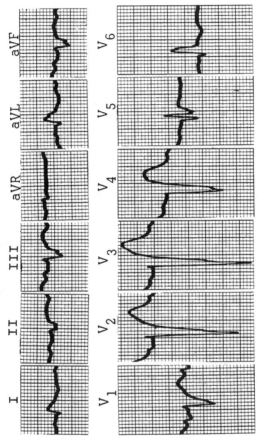

FIGURE 6–26 Complete LBBB with MI proved by autopsy. The ECG diagnosis of MI is based on the Q waves in leads I, aVL, V_5, and V_6. An autopsy performed 10 days later showed severe generalized atherosclerosis with total occlusion of the left circumflex artery. There was an extensive recent lateral wall MI in addition to a previous one. LVH also was present. (From Chou TC. Electrocardiography in Clinical Practice, 4th ed. Philadelphia: WB Saunders, 1996, p 181.)

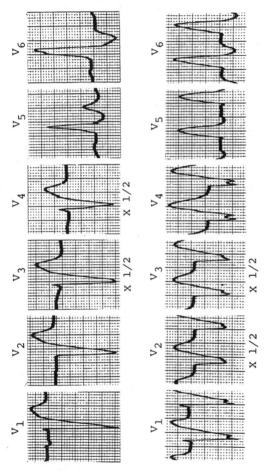

FIGURE 6–27 LBBB and MI. The patient was a 57-year-old man with a history of hypertension and coronary artery disease. The tracing on 2-7-69 was recorded after he developed CHF and experienced more frequent attacks of angina pectoris. It shows first-degree AV block, complete LBBB with a QRS duration of 0.18 second, and a digitalis effect. On 3-28-69, he developed severe substernal chest pain and episodes of ventricular tachycardia. The ECG shows the loss of R waves in leads V_3 and V_4 and the development of a small Q wave in lead V_5. The patient died 5 days later. At autopsy the heart weighed 1200 g with marked biventricular hypertrophy. Severe coronary artery disease was present, with a massive acute anterior MI. An old inferior MI and fatty degeneration and infiltration of the interventricular septum also were observed. (From Chou TC. Electrocardiography in Clinical Practice, 4th ed. Philadelphia: WB Saunders, 1996, p 182.)

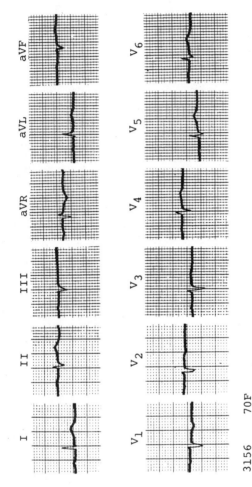

3156   70F

FIGURE 6–28 Myxedema heart disease. The patient is a 70-year-old woman with a 15-year history of myxedema. Symptoms and signs of myxedema recurred 1 year after she stopped taking her medication. She has no symptoms of coronary artery disease. The heart is not enlarged on radiographic examination. The ECG shows first-degree AV block. There is low voltage of the P waves and the QRS complexes with abnormal left axis deviation. The T waves are inverted in leads V_1 through V_3. (From Chou TC. Electrocardiography in Clinical Practice, 4th ed. Philadelphia: WB Saunders, 1996, p 270.)

- Constrictive pericarditis
- Myxedema (Fig. 6–28)
- Amyloidosis and other restrictive cardiomyopathy and diffuse myocardial disease
- Pleural effusion
- COPD

7

Atrial and Ventricular Hypertrophy

ATRIAL HYPERTROPHY

LEFT ATRIAL HYPERTROPHY

Diagnostic Criteria

- The P wave duration should be ≥ 0.12 second (3 small squares), and the P wave may be widely notched. These features are most apparent in lead 2 (Fig. 7–1).
- Downward terminal deflection of the P waves in V_1. The product of the depth of the terminal negative deflection in millimeters and the duration in seconds (the P terminal force) is ≥ 0.04 mm/s. The P terminal force is determined rapidly by observing the P wave in V_1. The P wave terminal negative duration equal to 1 small square and a depth of 1 small square (1 mm) yield a P terminal force of 0.04 mm/s (Figs. 7–1 and 7–2). These changes are observed in patients with left atrial enlargement or hypertrophy and in patients with an increase in left atrial pressure and volume. Thus the term *left atrial abnormality* is used by some cardiologists.

Causes

Left atrial hypertrophy is a common ECG finding. Causes of left atrial abnormality include

- Mitral stenosis.
- Mitral regurgitation.
- Left ventricular failure, in particular, acute pulmonary edema in which the abnormality may decrease or disappear after about 1 week of successful therapy.

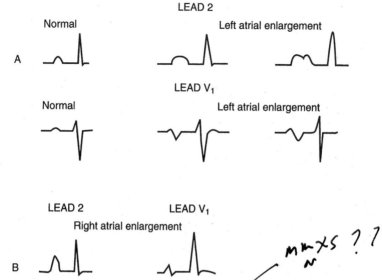

LEAD 2

Normal   Left atrial enlargement

A

LEAD V₁

Normal   Left atrial enlargement

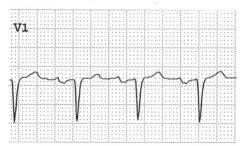

LEAD 2   LEAD V₁

Right atrial enlargement

mm×s ? ?

B

FIGURE 7–1   **A,** Left atrial enlargement: P wave duration ≥ 3 mm (0.12 second) in lead 2; in lead V₁ the negative component of the P wave occupies at least one small box = 1 mm × 0.04 = P terminal force > 0.04 mm/s (Fig. 7–2). **B,** Right atrial enlargement: lead 2 shows P amplitude ≥ 3 mm; in V₁ the first half of the P wave is positive and > 1 mm wide. (From Khan MG. On Call Cardiology. Philadelphia: WB Saunders, 1997, p 60.)

FIGURE 7–2   Lead V₁ shows typical P wave pattern of left atrial enlargement.

- Left ventricular hypertrophy; the atrium hypertrophies in response to altered left ventricular compliance.
- Aortic valve disease.

RIGHT ATRIAL HYPERTROPHY

Diagnostic Criteria

- The P wave is tall and peaked with a height > 2.5 mm in lead II, III, or aVF and is of normal duration (Fig. 7–3).

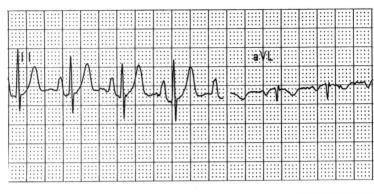

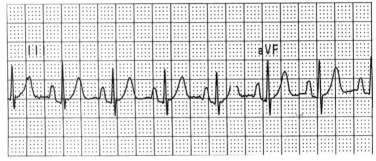

FIGURE 7–3 Leads II, III, and aVF show tall, peaked P waves greater than 2.5 mm.

- The positive component of the P wave in lead V_1 or V_2 is tall and peaked with a height > 1.5 mm.
- The P wave frontal axis is ≥ 75°.

Causes

Right atrial hypertrophy is an uncommon ECG finding; the causes of right atrial hypertrophy include

- Cor pulmonale.
- Pulmonary hypertension.
- Tricuspid hypertension.
- Tricuspid regurgitation.
- Right ventricular hypertrophy.

BILATERAL ATRIAL HYPERTROPHY

Bilateral enlargement is indicated by a large biphasic P wave in lead V_1, with the positive component > 1.5 mm and the initial terminal negative deflection reaching 1 mm in depth and ≥ 0.04 second in duration (Figs. 7–1 and 2–3).

VENTRICULAR HYPERTROPHY

LEFT VENTRICULAR HYPERTROPHY (LVH)

The genesis of the normal QRS complex is described in Chapter 3, and the genesis of the QRS complex in LVH is shown in Figure 7–4. In LVH the left atrium becomes hypertrophied to compensate for decreased compliance of the compromised left ventricle. Left atrial hypertrophy is an early ECG manifestation of LVH.

Diagnostic Criteria (Subjects Age ≥ 35 Years)

The QRS duration must be < 0.12 second.

1. **Sokolow-Lyon Voltage Criteria**
   - R wave in lead I + S wave in lead II or III > 25 mm.
   - R wave in aVL > 11 mm.
   - R wave in V_5 or V_6 > 26 mm.
   - R wave in V_5 or V_6 + S wave in V_1 or V_2 > 35 mm (Figs. 7–5 and 1–25).

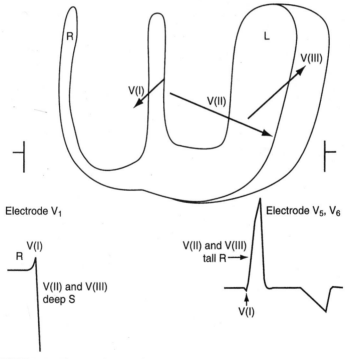

FIGURE 7–4 The contribution of vector II to the ECG features of LVH. The thicker the left ventricular muscle, the greater the magnitude of vector II, and therefore, the deep S wave in lead V_1 and tall R wave in leads V_5 and V_6. Note that the T wave has a gradual descending and a steep ascending limb "strain pattern." (From Khan MG. On Call Cardiology. Philadelphia: WB Saunders, 1997, p 78.)

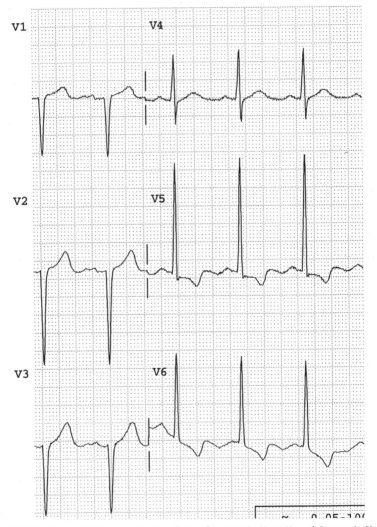

FIGURE 7–5   Marked increase in voltage of R wave in V_5 or V_6 and S wave in V_1 or $V_2 > 35$ mm. There is asymmetric ST segment depression and T wave inversion in V_5 and V_6, features typical of LVH.

Supporting Evidence

– Asymmetric ST segment depression and T wave inversion in V_5 and V_6: left ventricular strain pattern; the proximal descending limb of the inverted T wave has a slow descent, and the ascending limb rises steeply. These changes should be greater in V_5 and V_6 and less than in V_4 (Figs. 7–7 and 1–25). ST-T changes that are more prominent in V_3 and V_4 than in V_5 reflect ischemia.

– Left axis is supportive of LVH but is not necessary for the diagnosis.

– Onset of intrinsicoid deflection in V_5 or V_6 ≥ 0.05 second.

2. **Cornell Voltage**
   - S wave in V_3 and R wave in aVL > 28 mm in men or ≥ 20 mm in women.

3. **Author's Criteria (Subjects Age > 35 Years): 1 point = LVH**
   - S wave in V_1 or V_2 + R wave in V_5 or V_6 ≥ 35 mm = 1 point.
   - R wave in aVL + S wave in V_3 > 24 mm in men or > 18 mm in women = 1 point.
   - Left atrial enlargement = ½ point.
   - Asymmetric ST depression in V_5 and V_6 = ½ point.

4. **Romhilt-Estes Scoring System**
   - An R wave in the limb leads of ≥ 20 mm, an S wave in lead V_1 or V_2 ≥ 30 mm, or an R wave in lead V_5 or V_6 of > 30 mm = 3 points.
   - A P terminal force in lead V_1 of ≥ 0.04/s = 3 points.
   - ST-T wave changes (if not taking digoxin) = 3 points (taking digoxin = 1 point).
   - A left axis = 2 points.
   - A score of 4 points indicates probable LVH, and a score of 5 or more points indicates LVH.

Pitfalls in Diagnosis of LVH

- The preceding criteria do not apply in subjects younger than age 35 years because QRS voltage can be markedly increased in healthy young individuals (Fig. 7–6; see Table 1–1, p. 3).
- QRS voltage is increased by left anterior fascicular block.
- QRS voltage is higher in blacks than in whites.
- Conditions that decrease QRS voltage and that may mask the ECG signs of LVH include severe chronic obstructive pulmonary disease (COPD), pericardial effusion, large, old anterior infarcts, myxedema (Fig. 6–28), and heart muscle disease such as amyloidosis and scleroderma.

RIGHT VENTRICULAR HYPERTROPHY (RVH)

The QRS duration must be < 0.12 second; thus the diagnosis of RVH cannot be made accurately in the presence of right bundle branch block (RBBB) or Wolff-Parkinson-White (WPW) syndrome.

Diagnostic Criteria (Subjects Age > 30 Years)

Two or more of the following criteria are required for the diagnosis of RVH:

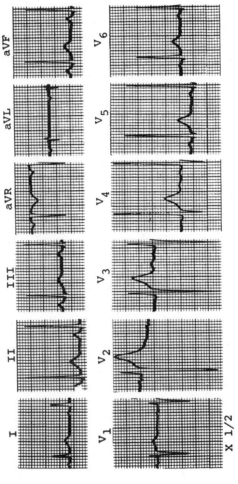

FIGURE 7–6 Normal young adult with high QRS voltage. The ECG was recorded from a healthy 22-year-old male medical student. R in V_5 + S in V_1 = 46 mm, and R in V_5 + S in V_2 = 49.5 mm. (From Chou TC. Electrocardiography in Clinical Practice, 4th ed. Philadelphia: WB Saunders, 1996, p 46.)

X 1/2

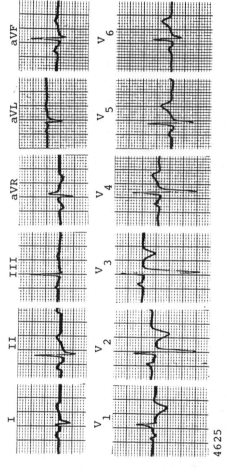

4 6 2 5

FIGURE 7–7 Severe mitral stenosis. The patient is a 47-year-old man with severe mitral stenosis proved at surgery. In the ECG the P waves are consistent with biatrial enlargement. The abnormal right axis deviation with an R/S ratio greater than 1 in lead V_1 and the T wave inversion in the right precordial leads are consistent with RVH. (From Chou TC. Electrocardiography in Clinical Practice, 4th ed. Philadelphia: WB Saunders, 1996, p 58.)

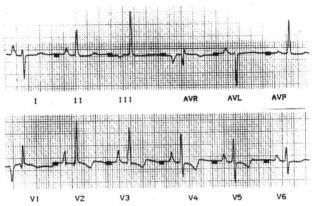

FIGURE 7–8   RVH. Q wave in V_1 suggests that the right ventricular pressure exceeds the left ventricular pressure. The left axis of the P wave and the prominent negative P wave in lead V_1 are unusual and most likely are due to a markedly enlarged right atrium projecting to the left and posteriorly. The prominent P waves in leads V_2 and V_3 are diagnostic of right atrial enlargement. (From Braunwald E. Heart Disease: A Textbook of Cardiovascular Medicine, 5th ed. Philadelphia: WB Saunders, 1997, p 146.)

- Right axis deviation of $\geq +110°$.
- Tall R wave in $V_1 > 7$ mm; S wave in $V_1 < 2$ mm; R/S ratio ≥ 1; R/S ratio in $V_1 > 1$ (Fig. 7–7); patient older than age 30 years (see Table 1–1, p. 3).
- S wave in V_5 or $V_6 \geq 2$ mm.
- qR pattern in V_1 (Fig. 7–8).

Supporting Evidence
- Onset of intrinsicoid deflection in $V_1 = 0.035$ to 0.055 second.
- ST-T strain pattern in V_1 through V_3 (Fig. 7–7).
- Right atrial enlargement.

Pitfalls in Diagnosis of RVH
RVH or right atrial enlargement are uncommon ECG diagnoses; refrain from making an ECG diagnosis of RVH in the presence of the following conditions:
- RBBB.
- WPW syndrome.
- True posterior myocardial infarction.
- In children (the preceding ECG findings can be a normal variant).
- Early transition; the R wave is increased in V_1 and V_2, but the R/S ratio in V_5 or V_6 is > 1.
- Dextroposition (see Table 1–3, p. 17).
- Hypertrophic cardiomyopathy: a tall R wave in V_1 with an R/S ratio > 1 may be observed.

8

T Waves

The T wave represents repolarization, the recovery period of the ventricles. As emphasized in Chapter 5, ST Segment Abnormalities, the skillful interpreter focuses on the ST segment and does not try to make diagnoses based on T wave changes. T wave changes are often nonspecific and should be interpreted always in the light of associated abnormalities of the ST segment and clinical findings. An algorithmic approach for the interpretation of T wave changes is depicted in Figure 8–1.

NORMAL DIRECTION OF T WAVE

- The T wave is always upright (positive) in leads I (1), II (2), and V_4 through V_6 (Figs. 8–2 and 8–3).
- The T wave is normally upright in lead aVF if the QRS complex is > 5 mm tall, but the T wave can be flat or inverted.
- The T wave is variable in leads III and aVL.
- The T wave is always inverted in aVR (Fig. 8–2).
- The T wave in V_1 is inverted in approximately 50% of women and in < 25% of men (Fig. 8–2).
- In women with persistent juvenile pattern the T wave is inverted in V_1 and V_2 and sometimes in V_3 (Fig. 8–4). This finding is common in black women.

ABNORMALITIES OF T WAVE

INVERTED T WAVE

- T wave inversion in leads I, II, and V_4 through V_6 is abnormal.
- If T wave inversion is accompanied by abnormal coving of the ST segment—horizontal or downsloping ST segment depression > 1 mm (Figs. 8–5 and 1–29)—a diagnosis of ischemia can be made with confidence.

STEP 8

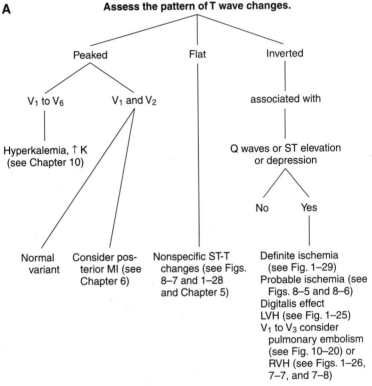

FIGURE 8–1   Method for rapid ECG interpretation. **A,** Step 8: Assessment of T wave changes.

STEP 8   *Continued*

B   **Assess the pattern of T wave changes.**

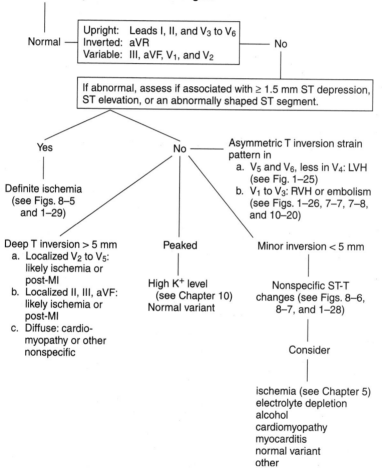

FIGURE 8–1 *Continued*   **B,** Step 8: Alternative methods.

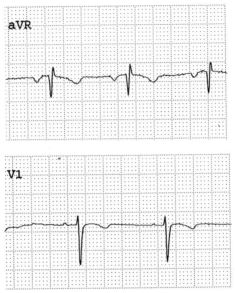

FIGURE 8–2 Shows normally occurring negative T waves in aVR and V₁.

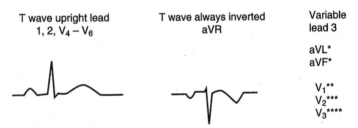

T wave upright lead 1, 2, V₄ – V₆	T wave always inverted aVR	Variable lead 3
		aVL* aVF*
		V₁** V₂*** V₃****

* = usually upright; can be inverted if R wave < 5 mm.

** = inverted in > 50% of women and < 20% of men who are > 30 years of age.

*** = usually upright; can be inverted with juvenile pattern.

**** = usually upright; rarely flat or biphasic in women or with juvenile pattern.

FIGURE 8–3 T wave, normal variability. (From Khan MG. On Call Cardiology. Philadelphia: WB Saunders, 1997, p 62.)

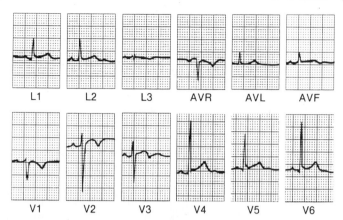

FIGURE 8–4   Normal tracing with juvenile T wave inversion in leads V_1 through V_3 and early repolarization manifested by ST segment elevation in leads I, II, aVF, and V_4 through V_6. (From Braunwald E. Heart Disease: A Textbook of Cardiovascular Medicine, 5th ed. Philadelphia: WB Saunders, 1997, p 138.)

- If T wave inversion is associated with ≤ 1 mm ST depression or an up-sloping depression, the finding is nonspecific (Fig. 8–6) and can be caused by a host of cardiac and noncardiac conditions.
- Isolated T wave inversion is nonspecific (Fig. 8–7A,B).

Diffuse, deep T wave inversion in the absence of ST segment elevation or significant depression is not diagnostic (Fig. 8–7A,B) and can be associated with

- Ischemia (Fig. 8–7C,D)
- Post myocardial infarction (MI) evolutionary changes
- Left ventricular hypertrophy (LVH) (Fig. 8–7C,D)
- Post Stokes-Adams attack
- Post supraventricular tachycardia or ventricular tachycardia
- Myocarditis
- Pericarditis
- Apical cardiomyopathy (giant T wave inversion)
- Pulmonary embolism
- Cardiomyopathies
- Primary or secondary cardiac tumors
- Cocaine abuse
- Alcohol abuse
- Electrolyte imbalance
- Subarachnoid hemorrhage (Fig. 8–8)
- Acute pancreatitis and gallbladder disease
- Pheochromocytoma
- Other causes

Symmetric T wave inversion is four times more common in women than it is in men. The interpretation of symmetric, deep T wave inversion as a sign of ischemia without considering other diagnoses is a common error.

Text continued on page 158

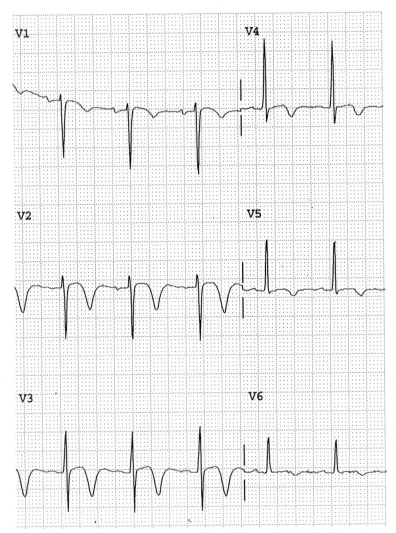

FIGURE 8–5   A, T wave inversion in V_2 through V_5 associated with abnormal curvature of the ST segment; likely caused by ischemia.

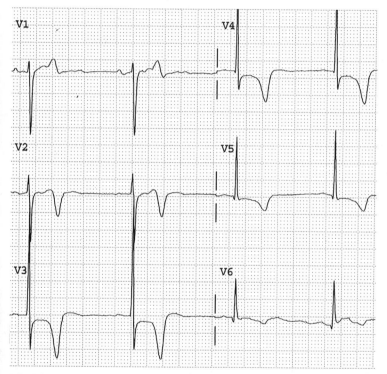

FIGURE 8–5 *Continued* **B,** Tracing from a 53-year-old woman with a 1-week history of unstable angina. Tracing taken in the absence of pain. Deep T wave inversion in V_2 through V_4. Note the abnormal coving of the ST segment and "hitched-up" ST segment in V_1 and V_2: definite ischemia.

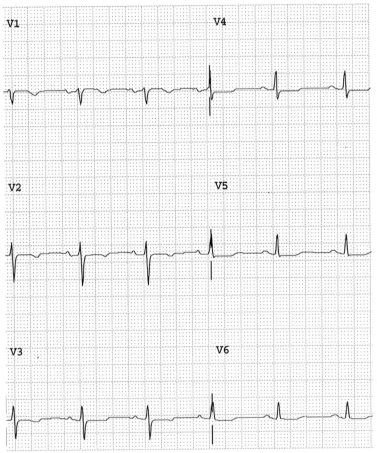

FIGURE 8–6 Minimal T wave inversion in V_2 through V_4 with < 1 mm ST depression: nonspecific ST-T changes; cannot exclude ischemia.

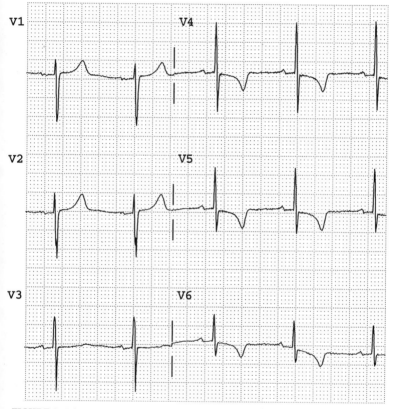

FIGURE 8–7   A, T wave inversion in V_4 through V_6; similar changes were observed in leads aVL, II, III, and aVF: nonspecific ST-T changes; cannot exclude ischemia.

Figure continued on following page

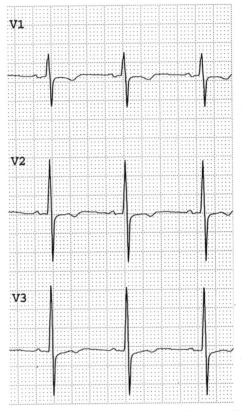

FIGURE 8–7 *Continued* **B,** Tracing from a 50-year-old man with no history of heart disease; nonspecific ST-T wave changes as seen from V₁ through V₃; the limb leads show no abnormality: borderline ECG.

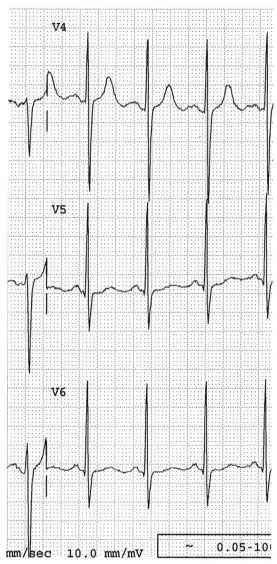

FIGURE 8–7 *Continued*   **C,** Voltage increase: probable LVH; compare to *D*.

Figure continued on following page

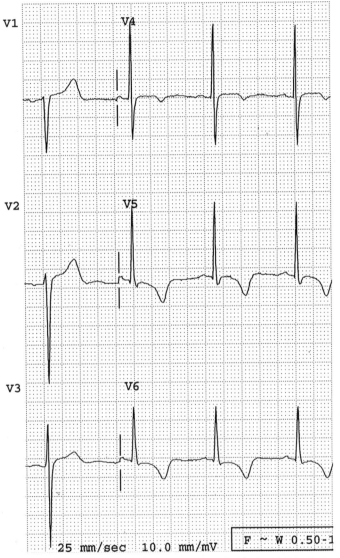

FIGURE 8–7 *Continued*   **D,** Same patient 12 hours later: The ST-T in V₄ through V₆, which was caused by ischemia, may have been interpreted incorrectly as LVH with "strain" pattern if *C* had not been available.

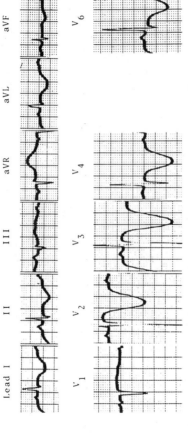

FIGURE 8–8 Patient with subarachnoid hemorrhage. ECG shows many of the findings frequently associated with central nervous system lesion. Careful autopsy examination revealed mild LVH and dilatation but no myocardial damage. (From Chou TC, Susilavorn B: Electrocardiographic changes in intracranial hemorrhage. J Eletrocardiol 1969;2:193. By permission.)

Minor T wave inversion not associated with significant ST segment changes can be caused by all of the conditions listed above and also by

- Hyperventilation.
- Postprandial: after a meal or cold drink the tracing normalizes in the fasting state.
- Normal variant: T wave inversion occurs in V_1 through V_3 in some young adults as a persistent juvenile pattern; this is more common in women (Fig. 8–4). Benign T wave inversion in V_4 through V_6 may be

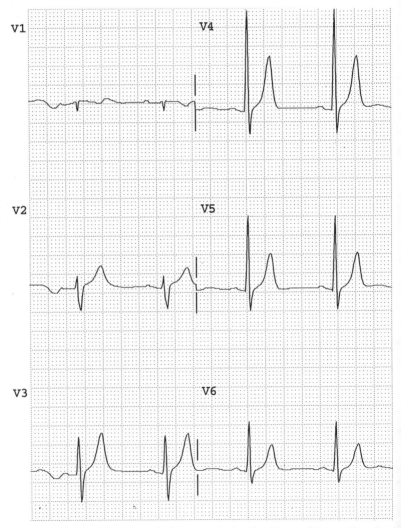

FIGURE 8–9 Prominent, peaked T waves in healthy 52-year-old man. Note the wide base as opposed to the narrow base T waves found in hyperkalemia.

observed in healthy young adults and may be associated with ST elevation as a normal variant (see Chapter 5).

- Mitral valve prolapse.
- Intraventricular conduction defects.
- Pneumothorax.
- Ventricular hypertrophy (see Chapter 7).

TALL T WAVES

The height of the normal T wave is usually < 5 mm in the limb leads and < 10 mm in any precordial lead. T waves that are > 6 mm in the limb leads or > 10 mm in the precordial leads may occur

- In V_2 through V_5 in some normal individuals. Note the base of normal peaked T waves is not narrow, as it is with hyperkalemia (Fig. 8–9). Occasionally peaked T waves may be associated with ST elevation occurring as a normal variant, commonly termed *repolarization changes* (see Chapters 1 and 5).
- With severe myocardial ischemia or acute MI (hyperacute T waves may occur).
- With hyperkalemia (see Chapter 10).
- With left ventricular overload as in severe mitral regurgitation.
- Occasionally with cerebrovascular accidents.

9

Electrical Axis and
Fascicular Block

ELECTRICAL AXIS

The electrical axis is discussed early and extensively in most books on ECG interpretation. Although the electrical axis is an important parameter that should be documented, it provides little or no assistance in the diagnosis of most cardiac conditions, in particular those that require specific therapy.

Determination of the electrical axis is useful mainly in the diagnosis of 4 of the 100 or more diagnoses made from ECG tracings:

1. **Left anterior fascicular block (hemiblock) (LAFB).**
2. **Right ventricular hypertrophy (RVH).** Right axis deviation is usually a feature. The electrical axis is of minor assistance in the diagnosis of left ventricular hypertrophy (LVH); left axis is not necessary for the diagnosis of LVH.
3. **Ventricular tachycardia (VT).** Some forms of VT are associated with left axis deviation or an axis in "no man's land," but right axis deviation may occur in some.
4. **Left posterior fascicular block** (see p. 170). Criteria for the diagnosis of left posterior fascicular block (LPFB) are inaccurate.

Figure 9–1 shows the vectoral genesis of the QRS complex and axis. The addition of all the vectors of ventricular depolarization produces one large mean QRS vector. The QRS axis represents the direction of the mean QRS vector in the frontal plane. The electrical axis is determined by using the hexaxial reference system, which was derived from the Einthoven equilateral triangle (Fig. 9–2).

Because of the minor contribution of the electrical axis to clinical cardiologic diagnosis, this topic is discussed late in this book and is relegated to step 9 in the 11-step method for rapid ECG diagnosis. See Figure 9–3,

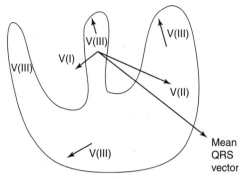

FIGURE 9–1 The mean QRS vector.

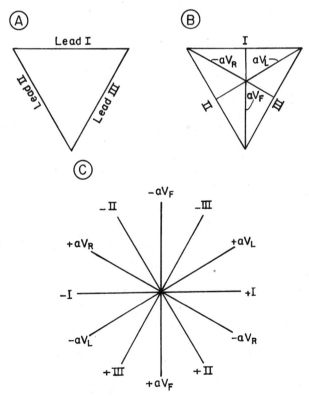

FIGURE 9–2 **A,** Einthoven's equilateral triangle formed by leads I, II, and III. **B,** The unipolar limb leads are added to the quilateral triangle. **C,** The hexaxial reference system derived from *B.* (From Chou TC. Electrocardiography in Clinical Practice, 4th ed. Philadelphia: WB Saunders, 1996, p 7.)

STEP 9

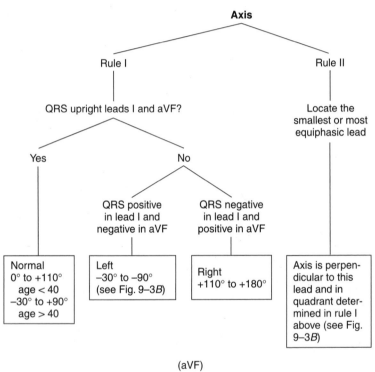

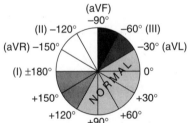

FIGURE 9–3 **A,** Method for rapid ECG interpretation. Step 9: Detection of the electrical axis. Leads are indicated in parentheses. See Table 9–1.

STEP 9   *Continued*

Axis	Lead I	aVF	II	III	aVR	aVL
Normal +45°				*		
Normal +60°						*
Left axis −45°			*			
−60°					*	
Right axis +150°			*			

*Most equiphasic lead.

FIGURE 9–3 *Continued*   **B,** See Table 9–1 and Figures 9–4 and 9–5.

TABLE 9–1   *Electrical Axis*

MOST EQUIPHASIC LEAD	LEAD PERPENDICULAR*	AXIS
		Leads I and aVF positive = Normal axis
III	aVR	Normal = +30°
aVL	II	Normal = +60°
		Lead I positive and aVF negative = Left axis
II	aVL (QRS positive)	Left = −30°
aVR	III (QRS negative)	Left = −60°
I	aVF (QRS negative)	Left = −90°
		Lead I negative and aVF positive = Right axis
aVR	III (QRS positive)	Right = +120°
II	aVL (QRS negative)	Right = +150°

*Lead perpendicular (at right angles) to the most equiphasic (isoelectric) lead usually has the tallest R or deepest S wave.

Table 9–1, and instructions given in Chapter 1 for the determination of the electrical axis.

- The range of the electrical axis in normal adults over the age of 40 is –30° to +90° (Fig. 9–3); for those under age 40, it is 0° to +105°. Normal children may have an axis of up to +110°. Most normal individuals have values between +30° and +75°.

LEFT AXIS DEVIATION (LAD)

An axis of –15° to –30° is sometimes termed *mild LAD,* and –45° to –90° is termed *marked LAD* (Fig. 9–4).

Causes

- Normal variation
- LAFB (hemiblock)
- Left bundle branch block (LBBB)
- LVH
- Mechanical shifts causing a horizontal heart; high diaphragm

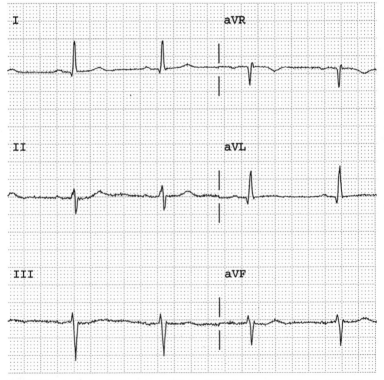

FIGURE 9–4   Left axis deviation –45°; lead II is the most equiphasic QRS; aVL is perpendicular and lies at –30°; aVR is the next most equiphasic; lead III is perpendicular at –60°; therefore the axis that lies between = –45° (see Fig. 9–3*B*).

- Some forms of VT
- Endocardial cushion defects

RIGHT AXIS DEVIATION (RAD)

Criteria for RAD in adults include
- Axis +101° to +180°.
- An axis of +105° to +120° is sometimes termed *mild RAD,* and an axis of +120° to +180° is termed *marked RAD* (Fig. 9–5).

Causes
- Normal variation
- RVH
- LPFB
- Lateral myocardial infarction (MI)
- Pulmonary embolism
- Dextrocardia
- Normal variants: mechanical shifts or emphysema causing a vertical heart

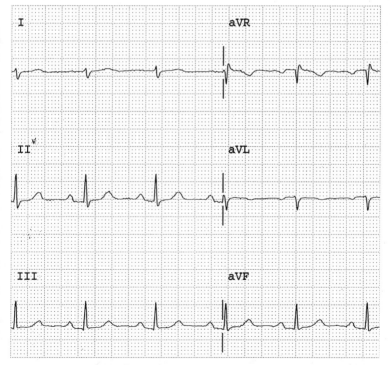

FIGURE 9–5 **A,** Right axis deviation; QRS axis +110°; lead I is the most equiphasic; aVF is perpendicular at +90°; aVR is the next most equiphasic with lead III being perpendicular at +120°; the exact axis lies somewhere between +90° and +120°, i.e., at +110°. Patient age > 40 years. *Figure continued on following page*

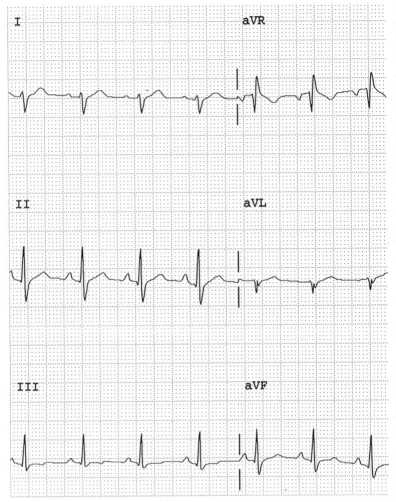

FIGURE 9–5 *Continued*   **B,** Right axis deviation. ECG from a 26-year-old healthy man.

LEFT ANTERIOR FASCICULAR BLOCK (HEMIBLOCK)

Figure 9–6 illustrates the division of the left bundle branch into anterior and posterior fascicles. The anterior fascicle traverses an anterosuperior course and ends at the base of the anterior papillary muscle. The anterior fascicle is thin and long, has a single blood supply, and is commonly damaged by ischemic disease fibrosis and other pathologic processes, resulting in LAFB. Rosenbaum initially called the block *left anterior hemiblock*, and because this term is easy to write, many cardiologist use it rather than LAFB.

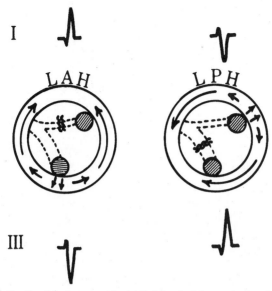

FIGURE 9–6 Hemiblock patterns in the limb leads: left anterior hemiblock (LAH) and left posterior hemiblock (LPH). The "anterior" papillary muscle is above and lateral to the "posterior" papillary muscle, and the two divisions of the left bundle branch course toward their respective papillary muscles. Thus, if the anterior division is blocked, initial electromotive forces are directed downward and to the right, inscribing a small q wave in leads I and aVL and an S wave in leads II, III, and aVF. The subsequent forces are directed mainly upward and to the left, writing an R wave in I and aVL and an S in II, III, and aVF, to produce a left axis deviation. In LPH the initial forces spread upward and to the left to write an R in I and aVL and a small q in II, III, and aVF while subsequent forces are directed downward and to the right to produce right axis deviation. (From Marriott JLH. Practical Electrocardiography, 8th ed. Baltimore: Williams & Wilkins, 1988, p 90.)

Criteria for Diagnosis

- LAD: −45° to −90° (preferably −60° to −90°).
- A small q wave, 0.5 to < 2 mm deep in lead I, qR in I (Fig. 9–7).
- A small r wave, 1 to 4 mm tall in lead III, rS in III.
- A normal QRS duration provided that right bundle branch block (RBBB) is absent. Other fascicles conduct normally; thus depolarization of the ventricles is not delayed.

Figure 9–6 shows how the ECG configuration of LAFB is derived. With block of the anterior fascicle, depolarization starts at the posterior papillary muscle and inferior wall and proceeds upward, superiorly and to the left to activate the left ventricular muscle mass that lies above the papillary muscle. Thus the electrical axis is directed strongly to the left at −60° to −90°. Because the electrical impulse originating from the posterior papillary muscle travels initially downward from endocardium to epicardium, it registers a small r wave of < 4 mm in lead III; the small impulse is directed away from lead I, and thus causes a small q wave in lead I. The current then travels upward to

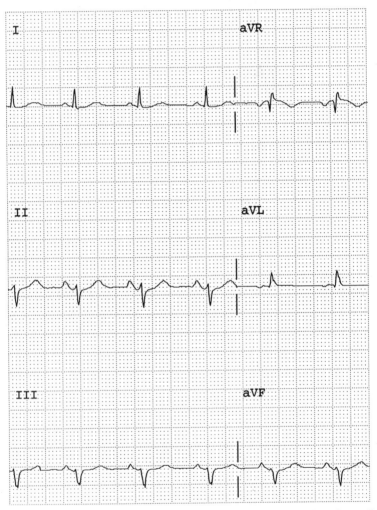

FIGURE 9–7   Left axis deviation –60°. There is a small q wave in lead I and a small r wave in lead III. These are the criteria for the diagnosis of LAFB: borderline ECG.

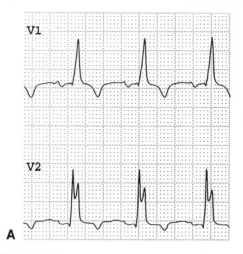

A

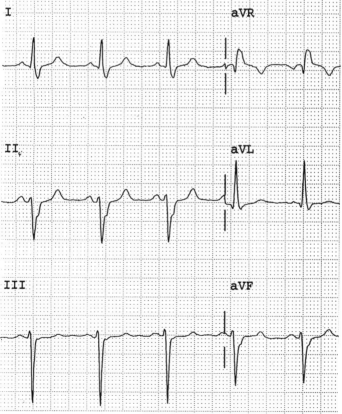

B

FIGURE 9–8   A, V leads from a patient with RBBB. **B,** Features of LAFB; the QRS complex is –75° with a small q wave in lead I and a small r wave in lead III in keeping with LAFB. Diagnosis: bifascicular block: RBBB and LAFB.

the left and causes an R wave in lead I and an S wave in lead III because electrical impulse travels away from the inferior leads (Figs. 9–4 and 9–6).

Causes and Pitfalls

- Acute or old MI. When LAFB occurs during acute inferior MI the initial small r wave caused by LAFB in leads II, III, and aVF masks the Q wave of infarction.
- Chronic ischemic heart disease without infarction is a common cause of LAFB.
- Cardiomyopathy and specific heart muscle disease.
- Hypertensive heart disease. LAFB lowers the QRS voltage in the precordial leads and may mask LVH; conversely LAFB increases QRS voltage in the limb leads and may mimic LVH.
- Chagas' disease.
- Myocarditis.
- A "normal" finding in approximately 1% of men over age 40.

LEFT POSTERIOR FASCICULAR BLOCK

LPFB or posterior hemiblock occurs rarely because the posterior bundle is thick and short and has a double blood supply. The fascicle runs to the base of the posterior papillary muscle (Fig. 9–6). The diagnosis can be made only after excluding RVH and chronic obstructive pulmonary disease (COPD). Criteria for the diagnosis of LPFB are

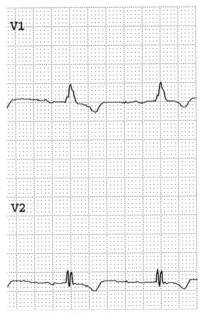

FIGURE 9–9   Tracing of a patient with RBBB and LPFB: bifascicular block. See page 171 for limb leads.

- RAD +120° to +180°
- A small r wave < 4 mm in lead I; an S wave in lead I.
- A small q wave in lead III.
- A normal QRS duration.
- RVH or cor pulmonale, COPD, a vertical heart, and other causes of RAD must be absent; thus a confident diagnosis of LPFB is not often made.

BIFASCICULAR BLOCK

- The combination of LAFB and RBBB occurs commonly (Fig. 9–8) but rarely progresses to serious block; thus, pacing is rarely required.
- The combination of LPFB and RBBB occurs rarely (Fig. 9–9).

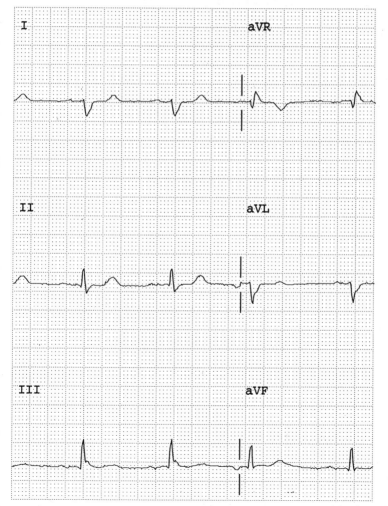

FIGURE 9–9 *Continued* See legend on opposite page.

10

Miscellaneous Conditions

After there has been a methodical assessment of the P waves, the QRS duration for bundle branch blocks (LBBB, RBBB), the ST segment, Q waves, hypertrophy, and electrical axis, an assessment for miscellaneous conditions is appropriate. A search for miscellaneous conditions is logically performed at step 10 (Fig. 10–1).

The ECG may reveal clues to the diagnosis of 12 or more miscellaneous conditions:

- Acute pericarditis
- Long QT interval
- Hypokalemia
- Hyperkalemia
- Digitalis toxicity
- Dextrocardia
- Electrical alternans
- Electronic pacing
- Pulmonary embolism (the ECG is not diagnostic)
- Hypothermia and hyperthermia
- Hypercalcemia and hypocalcemia

PERICARDITIS

DIAGNOSTIC CRITERIA

- **Stage 1:** Widespread ST segment elevation, generally upwardly concave in all leads except aVR and occasionally V_1. ST segment elevation may persist for a few days (Figs. 10–2 and 1–33). Reciprocal ST seg-

STEP 10   **Miscellaneous conditions**

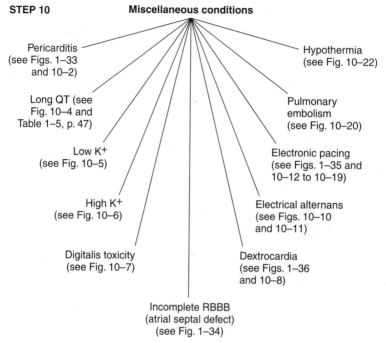

FIGURE 10–1   Method for rapid ECG interpretation. Step 10: Assess for miscellaneous conditions.

ment depression occurs in aVR and sometimes in V_1 (Fig. 10–1). PR segment depression generally occurs in all leads except aVR and occasionally V_1.

- **Stage 2:** A few days later the ST and PR segments become normal (isoelectric); the T wave remains normal or may be decreased in amplitude and may become flattened.
- **Stage 3:** After normalization of the ST segment, diffuse T wave inversion occurs.
- **Stage 4:** Lasts from days to weeks; the T waves normalize; rarely do they remain inverted.

OTHER CLUES SUGGESTIVE OF ACUTE PERICARDITIS

- Early PR segment depression, in particular in leads II, aVF, and V_4 through V_6.
- Sinus tachycardia may be the only finding if ST segment elevation has resolved and the T waves remain normal.
- Electrical alternans usually involves the QRS complex. Total alternans with involvement of the P, QRS, and T waves may occur with cardiac tamponade.
- Low voltage QRS may occur when pericardial fluid accumulates.

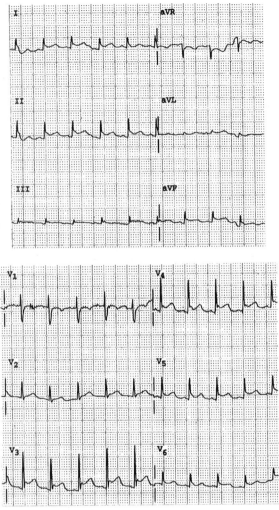

FIGURE 10–2   Widespread ST segment elevation, generally upwardly concave in all leads except aVR and V$_1$; acute pericarditis. (From Khan MG. Heart Disease Diagnosis and Therapy. Baltimore: Williams & Wilkins, 1996, p 479.)

LONG QT INTERVAL

- The QT interval indicates the total duration of ventricular systole. A prolonged QT interval represents delayed repolarization of the ventricles and predisposes to reentrant arrhythmias, such as torsades de pointes (see Chapter 11, p. 246, Fig. 11–43).
- As a rough guide, the QT interval should be less than half the preceding RR interval at heart rates of 60 to 100 beats per minute (bpm).

- The QT interval varies with heart rate, and several formulas have been used to provide a corrected QT interval (QTc).
- The QTc also has limitations because of difficulties and exact measurements. Because it is difficult sometimes to define the end of the T wave, the measurement is often inaccurate, particularly when a U wave merges with the T. Thus in clinical practice, assess the QT interval mainly for excessive prolongation: use a lead that does not show a U wave (Figs. 10–3 and 10–4).
- See Table 1–5, page 47, for a clinically useful approximation of QT intervals.

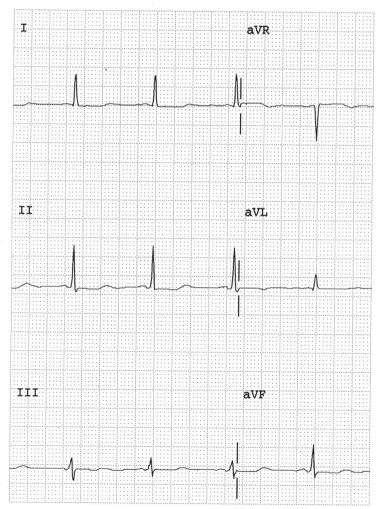

FIGURE 10–3   QT interval 0.46 second; the heart rate is 67 bpm. The normal range of a QT interval at a heart rate of 67 to 100 bpm is 0.33 to 0.42 second (see Table 1–5, p. 47).

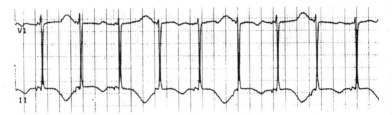

FIGURE 10–4 The QT interval is prolonged, measuring approximately 600 ms, with T wave alternans. The tracing was recorded in a patient with chronic renal disease shortly after dialysis. (From Braunwald E. Heart Disease: A Textbook of Cardiovascular Medicine, 5th ed. Philadelphia: WB Saunders, 1997, p 138.)

A **prolonged QT interval** may be caused by the following:

- Drugs
  - Class 1 antiarrhythmics: disopyramide, procainamide, and quinidine
  - Class 3 antiarrhythmics: amiodarone and sotalol
  - Tricyclic antidepressants
  - Phenothiazines
  - Astemizole
  - Terfenidine
  - Adenosine
  - Antibiotics: erythromycin and other macrolides
  - Antifungal agents
  - Pentamidine, chloroquine
- Ischemic heart disease
- Cerebrovascular disease
- Rheumatic fever
- Myocarditis
- Mitral valve prolapse
- Electrolyte abnormalities
- Hypocalcemia
- Hypothyroidism
- Liquid protein diets
- Organophosphate insecticides
- Congenital prolonged QT syndrome

A **short QT interval** is not of great concern and occurs rarely with the following:

- Hypercalcemia, a feature of malignancy and hyperparathyroidism
- Digitalis intoxication

HYPOKALEMIA

- Progressive ST segment depression: normally a small U wave has the same polarity as the T wave; when the serum potassium level falls to < 3.5 mEq/L, the amplitude of the T wave decreases.
- A marked increase in U wave amplitude: the U wave becomes taller than the T wave: with serum potassium < 1.5 mEq/L, the T and the U

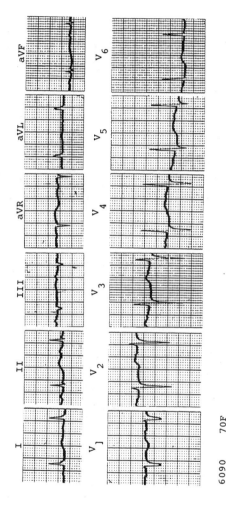

6090   70F

FIGURE 10-5 Hypokalemia produced by diuretics. The serum potassium level was 2.7 mEq/L; sodium, 124 mEq/L; and calcium 9.2 mg/dl. The ECG shows diffuse ST segment depression, T wave flattening, and prominent U waves. The prominent U waves may be mistaken for T waves. (From Chou TC. Electrocardiography in Clinical Practice, 4th ed. Philadelphia: WB Saunders, 1996, p 539.)

177

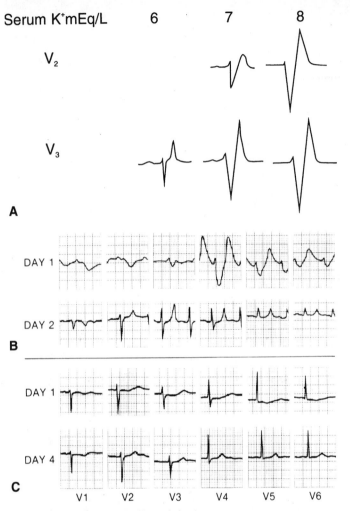

FIGURE 10–6 **A,** ECG signs of hyperkalemia.

- $K^+ > 5.7$ mEq/L: Earliest signs are T wave peaked, narrow base ("tented"); PR interval may be prolonged.
- $K^+ > 7$ mEq/L: P wave flat or absent; QRS widens; prominent S wave.
- $K^+ > 8$ mEq/L: S wave becomes wider and deeper and moves steeply into the T wave; there is virtually no isoelectric ST segment; occasionally ST segment elevation.

B, ECG changes in hyperkalemia. On day 1, at a K^+ level of 8.6 mEq/L, the P wave is no longer recognizable and the QRS complex is diffusely prolonged. Initial and terminal QRS delay is characteristic of K^+-induced intraventricular conduction and is best illustrated in leads V_2 and V_6. On day 2, at a K^+ level of 5.8 mEq/L, the P wave is recognizable with a PR interval of 0.24 second; the duration of the QRS complex is approximately 0.10 second; and the T waves are characteristically "tented." **C,** ECG changes in hypokalemia. On day 1, at a K^+ level of 1.5 mEq/L, the T and U waves are merged. The U wave is prominent and the QU interval prolonged. On day 4, at a K^+ level of 3.7 mEq/L, the tracing is normal. (*A* from Khan MG. Medical Diagnosis and Therapy. Philadelphia: Lea & Febiger, 1994, p 671. *B* and *C* from Braunwald E. Heart Disease: A Textbook of Cardiovascular Medicine, 5th ed. Philadelphia: WB Saunders, 1997, p 141.)

wave may become fused. The changes are seen best in leads V_2 through V_5 (Figs. 10–5 and 10–6C).
- ST segment depression.
- An increase in the QRS duration.
- Slight prolongation of the PR interval.

HYPERKALEMIA

- Mild hyperkalemia: at serum potassium < 6.5 mEq/L the P wave widens; tall, peaked, narrow-base, "tented" T waves in many leads (Fig. 10–6B); first-degree AV block.
- Severe hyperkalemia: at serum potassium > 6.5 mEq/L, marked widening of the second portion of the QRS complex, which may show notching or slurring, and thus the wide QRS merges with the tall, tented T waves; the ST segment may be elevated (Fig. 10–6).
- High-degree AV block: disappearance of P waves.
- Ventricular tachycardia (VT), ventricular fibrillation (VF), or idioventricular rhythm.

DIGITALIS TOXICITY

- Digitalis effect revealed by the ECG does not imply toxicity and is suggested by the following:
    - Sagging ST segment depression with upward concavity
    - Decreased amplitude of T wave, which may be biphasic
    - Shortening of the QT interval
    - Prolonged PR interval; first-degree AV block
    - Increased amplitude of the U wave
- Digitalis toxicity is suggested by the occurrence of almost any type of arrhythmia or conduction defect with the exception of bundle branch block: common arrhythmias include the following:
    - Excitant disturbances: ventricular premature beats (VPBs), especially bigeminy and multifocal VPBs; atrial tachycardia; AV junctional tachycardia; accelerated junctional rhythm; VT; bidirectional tachycardia; VF
    - Suppressant disturbances: sinus bradycardia, first-degree AV block, second-degree AV block, Mobitz type I (Wenckebach) block, complete AV block
    - Combined disturbances: atrial tachycardia with AV block (paroxysmal atrial tachycardia [PAT] with block); regular, accelerated junctional rhythm in the presence of atrial fibrillation (Fig. 10–7)

DEXTROCARDIA: TRUE DEXTROCARDIA (WITH SITUS INVERSUS)

- In lead I the P, QRS, and T waves are inverted or upside down (Fig. 10–8).
- Leads aVR and aVL are reversed; thus prominent negative deflections are recorded in aVL with positive deflections in aVR.

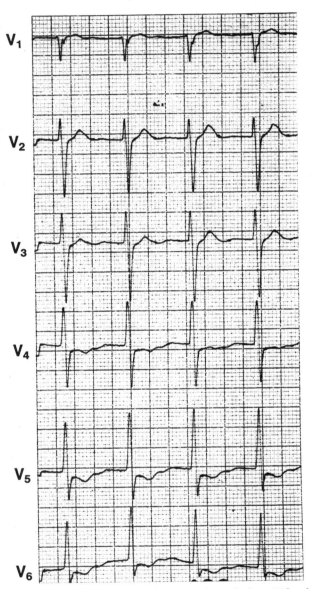

FIGURE 10-7   Atrial fibrillation with junctional tachycardia (rate: 95 bpm) due to digitalis toxicity. Note the absolute regularity of the rhythm. (From Wellens JJH. The ECG in Emergency Decision Making. Philadelphia: WB Saunders, 1992, p 147.)

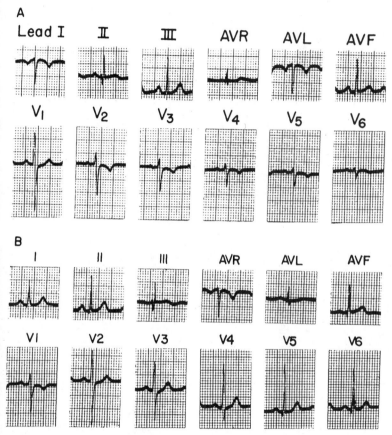

FIGURE 10–8   Mirror-image dextrocardia with sinus inversus. The patient is a 15-year-old girl. There is no evidence of organic heart disease. **A,** Tracing recorded with the conventional electrode placement. **B,** Tracing obtained with the left and right arm electrodes reversed. The precordial lead electrodes also were relocated in the respective mirror-image positions on the chest. The tracing is within normal limits. (From Chou TC. Electrocardiography in Clinical Practice, 4th ed. Philadelphia: WB Saunders, 1996, p 313.)

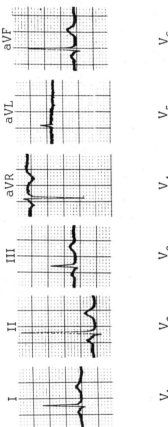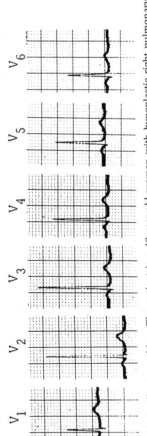

FIGURE 10–9 Dextroposition. The patient is a 40-year-old woman with hypoplastic right pulmonary artery and right lung, probably of congenital origin. The heart and mediastinum are displaced to the right chest. In the ECG the limb leads are normal except for a relatively large R wave in lead II and S wave in lead aVR. The precordial leads show tall R waves in leads V_1 through V_3; the amplitude of the R waves decreases from V_2 through V_6. (From Chou TC. Electrocardiography in Clinical Practice, 4th ed. Philadelphia: WB Saunders, 1996, p 314.)

- Lead II represents the usual lead III and vice versa.
- Lead aVF is unaffected.
- Decreased R wave amplitude from leads V_1 through V_6. V_1 is the equivalent of usual V_2 and vice versa; leads V_3 and V_4 are the equivalent of the usual V_{3R} and V_{4R}.
- Repeat ECG with a reversal of the right and left arm leads. Placement of the V leads in the equivalent positions on the right side of the chest is necessary for accurate interpretation of the ECG.
- Incorrect arm lead placement: reversal of the arm leads can produce similar recordings in I, aVR, and aVL but not in V_1 through V_6. A tip off to this error is the marked dissimilarity of the record in leads I and V_6.
- Isolated dextrocardia without situs inversus invariably is associated with complicated cardiac malformations and is rarely seen in adults.
- In dextroversion the heart is rotated to the right side of the chest, but the heart retains its normal configuration. The left atrium and ventricle remain to the left.
- In dextroposition the heart is displaced to the right by lung disease. The ECG is normal, but R waves are prominent in V_1 through V_3 and decrease in amplitude from V_2 through V_6 (Fig. 10–9).

ELECTRICAL ALTERNANS

- Regular alternation in the amplitude, direction, or configuration of the QRS complexes in any or all leads (Fig. 10–10). The RR intervals remain unchanged (regular).
- Total electrical alternans refers to involvement of the P, QRS, and T waves and occasionally the U wave.

CAUSES

- Alternans of the QRS complex is a rare finding in patients with cardiac tamponade and occurs in some patients with a large pericardial effusion, particularly with malignancy.
- Total electrical alternans is almost diagnostic of cardiac tamponade, although it occurs in < 10% of cases of tamponade and may be associated with a "swinging heart" on echocardiography.
- Severe coronary artery and hypertrophic heart disease is a rare cause.
- Supraventricular tachycardia with a very rapid ventricular rate, mainly occurring in patients with Wolff-Parkinson-White (WPW) syndrome (orthodromic) reentrant tachycardia (Fig. 10–11).

ELECTRONIC PACING

VENTRICULAR PACING

- The pacemaker impulse, a sharp narrow spike, is followed by a QRS complex of different morphology than the intrinsic QRS. With right

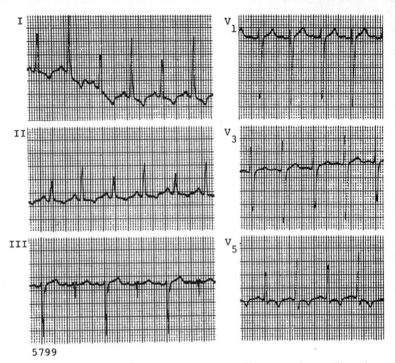

FIGURE 10–10 Electrical alternans in postpericardiotomy syndrome. The patient is a 30-year-old man who developed pericarditis and pericardial effusion 3 weeks after aortic valve surgery. In the ECG, in addition to the alternation of the QRS complex, T wave alternans can be seen in lead III. (From Chou TC. Electrocardiography in Clinical Practice, 4th ed. Philadelphia: WB Saunders, 1996, p 251.)

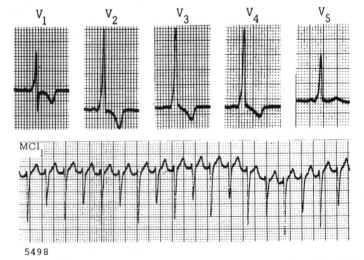

FIGURE 10–11 Electrical alternans during supraventricular tachycardia (orthodromic AV reentrant tachycardia). The patient is a 23-year-old woman with type A Wolff-Parkinson-White syndrome without other evidence of organic heart disease. Alternation of the QRS complex is seen during the tachycardia. (From Chou TC. Electrocardiography in Clinical Practice, 4th ed. Philadelphia: WB Saunders, 1996, p 253.)

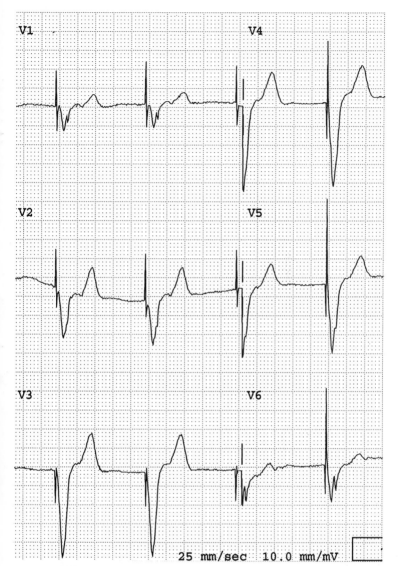

FIGURE 10–12 Electronic pacemaker, ventricular capture; rate = 60 bpm. No further analysis is attempted because of pacemaker rhythm.

ventricular pacing the QRS complex is similar to that of left bundle branch block (LBBB) (Fig. 10–12).

- With left ventricular epicardial myocardial pacing the QRS shows a right bundle branch block (RBBB) morphology.
- Pacemakers in a "unipolar pacing mode" cause a larger amplitude spike than that of bipolar pacing.
- Demonstrate inhibition of the pacemaker output in response to the intrinsic QRS.

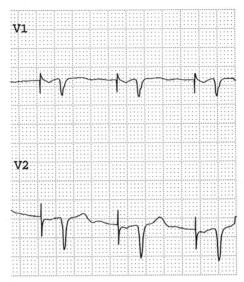

FIGURE 10–13 Electronic pacemaker, atrial pacing; rate = 70 bpm.

Ventricular Demand Pacing (VVI)

Output is inhibited by sensed ventricular signal.

ATRIAL PACING

Pacemaker spike is followed by P wave and narrow paced QRS complexes in response to paced atrial beats (Fig. 10–13).

Atrial Demand Pacing (AAI)

Output is inhibited by sensed atrial signal.

AV SEQUENTIAL PACING

- Atrial followed by ventricular pacing (Fig. 10–14).
- Could be pacing in both atrium and ventricle; senses R waves only: DVI pacing mode.
- Pacing and senses both atrium and ventricle: DDD mode; synchronizes with atrial activity and paces ventricle after preset AV interval (Fig. 10–15).
- Output is inhibited by sensed atrial signal (AAI) and by sensed ventricular signal (VVI), but tracking of atrial rate by ventricular sensing does not occur: DDI pacing mode.
- Fixed rate (asynchronous) atrial and ventricular pacing at specific AV interval: DOO pacing mode.

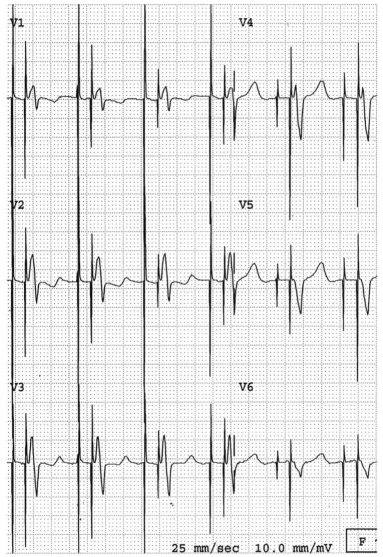

FIGURE 10–14 Electronic pacemaker, ventricular capture; rate = 72 bpm; AV sequential pacemaker.

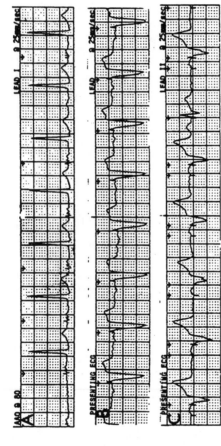

FIGURE 10–15 Different modes of pacemaker function are shown. **A**, AOO, fixed rate atrial pacing. Note narrow paced QRS complexes in response to paced atrial beats. **B**, VDD, the pacemaker senses the atrium and the ventricle and paces the ventricle. Each spontaneous P wave is followed by a paced ventricular complex. **C**, DDD pacing; the pacemaker senses and paces in the atrium and the ventricle. The sixth complex of this strip represents a spontaneous P wave that conducts to the ventricle, resulting in a narrow QRS complex with the pacing spike occurring in the ventricular refractory period. Arrows indicate pacing stimulus artefacts. (From Saksena S. In: Khan MG. Heart Disease Diagnosis and Therapy. Baltimore: Williams & Wilkins, 1996, p 584.)

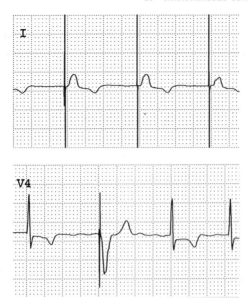

FIGURE 10–16   Electronic pacemaker, demand mode; ventricular capture rate = 75 bpm. Note the spontaneous beat in V_4 is followed by sensing and pacemaker capture at the appropriate interval, which is equal to that shown in lead I.

PACEMAKER MALFUNCTION

Undersensing Malfunction

For pacemaker in the inhibited mode, undersensing is diagnosed on ECG by a pacemaker spike at an inappropriately short interval after a spontaneous (intrinsic) event, i.e., a failure of the pacemaker to be inhibited by an appropriate intrinsic atrial or ventricular depolarization (QRS). Figure 10–16 shows accurate sensing. With sensing malfunction the pacemaker operates like a fixed-rate pacemaker; the spontaneous intrinsic QRS complexes are not sensed (Fig. 10–17).

Pacing Malfunction

- Not firing: failure of appropriate pacemaker output (Fig. 10–18).
- Slowing: an increase in stimulus intervals over the programmed intervals. The battery power failure is indicated by a decrease of the pacing rate (Fig. 10–19).

PULMONARY EMBOLISM (PE)

The ECG findings are nonspecific; more important, their transient occurrence should heighten clinical suspicion of PE:

- Sinus tachycardia.

Text continued on page 196

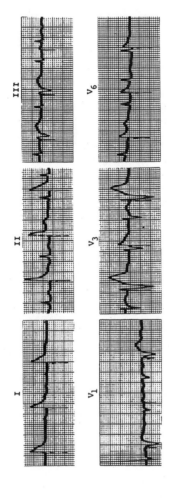

570909 64F

FIGURE 10–17 Ventricular demand pacemaker (VVI) with sensing malfunction. The pacemaker operates like a fixed-rate pacemaker. The spontaneous ventricular beats are not sensed. The spontaneous rhythm is atrial fibrillation. (From Chou TC. Electrocardiography in Clinical Practice, 4th ed. Philadelphia: WB Saunders, 1996, p 613.)

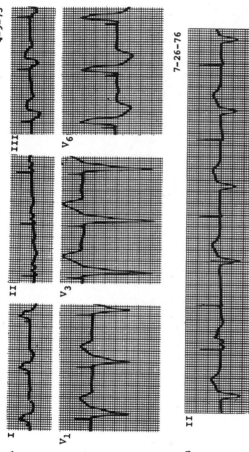

4-9-73

I II III

V₁ V₃ V₆

7-26-76

II

FIGURE 10–18 Right and left ventricular pacemakers and pacemaker malfunction. These tracings were obtained from the same patient. **A,** Tracing recorded when the patient had a transvenous right ventricular demand pacemaker that was functioning properly. Because there are no spontaneous beats, the demand function of the pacemaker cannot be demonstrated. **B,** Tracing showing intermittent pacing failure. The first QRS complex is a spontaneous beat. The second complex is pacemaker induced. The next pacemaker spike appears prematurely and is not followed by ventricular depolarization. A pseudo fusion beat follows. None of the last three pacemaker stimuli captures the ventricle. The sensing function of the pacemaker appears intact. The pacing malfunction was found to be the result of broken lead. (From Chou TC. Electrocardiography in Clinical Practice, 4th ed. Philadelphia: WB Saunders, 1996, p 617.)

Figure continued on following page

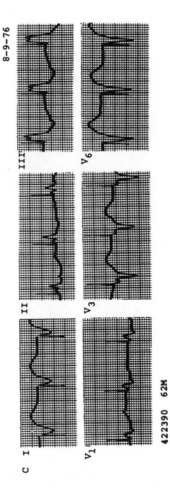

8-9-76

422390   62M

FIGURE 10–18   C, Tracing recorded after the patient received an epicardial left ventricular pacemaker. (From Chou TC. Electrocardiography in Clinical Practice, 4th ed. Philadelphia: WB Saunders, 1996, p 617.)

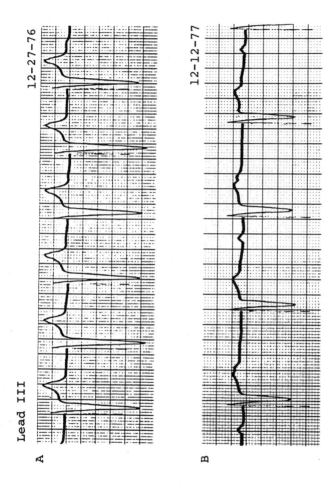

FIGURE 10-19 Battery failure. The battery power failure is indicated by a decrease of the pacing rate from 70 to 47 bpm. (From Chou TC. Electrocardiography in Clinical Practice, 4th ed. Philadelphia: WB Saunders, 1996, p 616.)

193

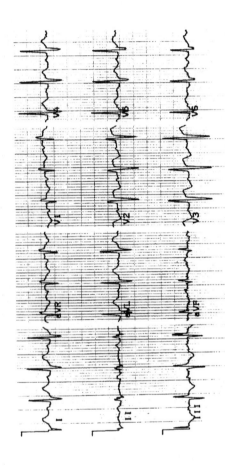

FIGURE 10–20 Acute massive pulmonary embolus with the characteristic S_1Q_3 pattern and the more common but nonspecific changes including incomplete RBBB and ST segment elevation in leads V_1 through V_3 with terminal T wave inversion. (From Braunwald E. Heart Disease: A Textbook of Cardiovascular Medicine, 5th ed. Philadelphia: WB Saunders, 1997, p 118.)

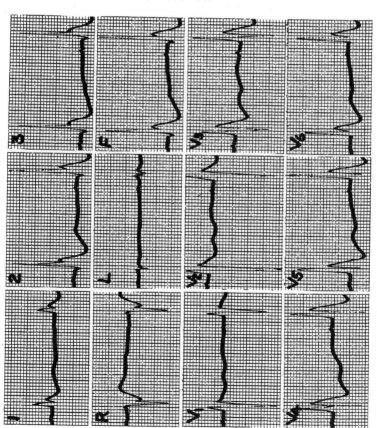

FIGURE 10-21 Hypothermia. Note marked elevation of the J deflection maximal in midprecordial leads. (From Marriott JLH. Practical Electrocardiography, 8th ed. Baltimore: Williams & Wilkins, 1988, p 522.)

195

- Symmetrical T wave inversion; strain pattern in leads V_1 through V_3 or V_4.
- ST depression may occur in leads I, II, and V_3 through V_6.
- S_1, Q_3; S_1, Q_3, T_3 pattern (Fig. 10–20).
- Incomplete or complete RBBB pattern.
- Q waves in leads V_1, III, and aVF but not in lead II.
- Qr in V_1.
- ST segment elevation in leads V_1 through V_2 or V_3, aVR, and III (Fig. 10–20).
- ST segment depression in V_3 through V_5 or V_6 because of associated myocardial ischemia.
- S_1, S_2, S_3 pattern.
- Arrhythmias that include premature beats, atrial flutter or atrial fibrillation, VF.
- Right atrial enlargement.
- Right axis deviation.

In the presence of submissive PE the ECG may show no significant abnormality. With massive PE causing syncope, cardiogenic shock, or acute right-sided heart failure, at least one of the preceding ECG changes usually occurs.

HYPOTHERMIA

- All intervals, PR, RR, QRS, and QT, may lengthen.
- Elevated "T waves" (Osborn waves) appear (Fig. 10–21); the start of the ST segment especially in V_3 and V_4 is elevated, hitched-up, representing distortion of early repolarization.
- Atrial fibrillation occurs often with temperatures below 32° C.

11

Arrhythmias

ATRIAL PREMATURE BEATS (APBs)

ECG Diagnostic Points

- An atrial premature P wave has a morphology different from that of the sinus P wave (Fig. 11–1).
- The premature P is usually followed by a QRS complex similar to that with the normally conducted sinus beat. The premature P wave may be unrecognizable because it is hidden in the preceding T wave, hence the admonition "search the T for the P" (Figs. 11–2 and 11–3).
- The PR interval of an APB is > 0.11 second; if the P wave is inverted in leads II, III, and aVF the PR should be > 0.11 second to distinguish an APB from a junctional premature beat (JPB).
- Early occurring APBs may trigger atrial tachycardia (Fig. 11–2), atrial flutter, or atrial fibrillation.
- APBs that follow every sinus beat cause atrial bigeminy (Fig. 11–1).
- The atrial premature P wave may not be conducted, resulting in a pause (Fig. 11–3). Nonconducted APBs are the most common cause of pauses; if the premature P waves are not identified, the rhythm may be misinterpreted as sinus bradycardia.
- If the APB traverses the atrioventricular (AV) junction at a time when one of the bundle branches is still refractory, aberrant ventricular conduction may occur. The QRS is wide and resembles a ventricular premature beat (VPB) (Fig. 11–2C). Examination of the preceding T wave may reveal a deformity caused by a P′ wave stuck on the T wave as shown in Figure 11–2C. Also, a postectopic cycle that is less than compensatory points to atrial ectopy with aberration.
- Multiple APBs may cause an irregularly irregular pulse.

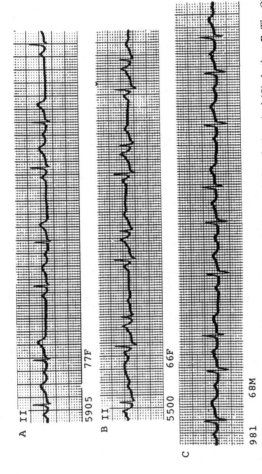

FIGURE 11–1 Premature atrial beats with bigeminal (**A** and **B**) and trigeminal (**C**) rhythm. **B,** The QRS complex of the premature atrial beats shows aberrant ventricular conduction. (From Chou TC. Electrocardiography in Clinical Practice, 4th ed. Philadelphia: WB Saunders, 1996, p 344.)

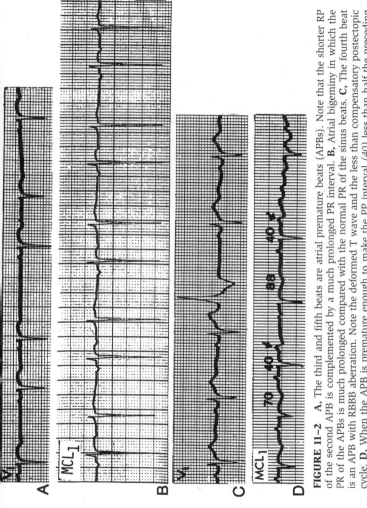

FIGURE 11-2 **A,** The third and fifth beats are atrial premature beats (APBs). Note that the shorter RP of the second APB is complemented by a much prolonged PR interval. **B,** Atrial bigeminy in which the PR of the APBs is much prolonged compared with the normal PR of the sinus beats. **C,** The fourth beat is an APB with RBBB aberration. Note the deformed T wave and the less than compensatory postectopic cycle. **D,** When the APB is premature enough to make the PP interval (*40*) less than half the preceding PP interval (*88*), an atrial tachyarrhythmia is triggered. (From Marriott JLH. Practical Electrocardiography, 8th ed. Baltimore: Williams & Wilkins, 1988, p 151.)

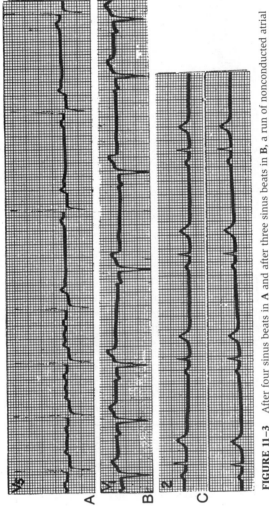

FIGURE 11–3 After four sinus beats in **A** and after three sinus beats in **B**, a run of nonconducted atrial bigeminy develops. Note in each strip the subtle deformity of the T wave compared with the preceding T waves, due to superimposed P' waves. In **C** the T waves look a little too pointed for natural T waves; but when no previous T waves are available for comparison, it is impossible to diagnose the atrial bigeminy. (From Marriott JLH. Practical Electrocardiography, 8th ed. Baltimore: Williams & Wilkins, 1988, p 150.)

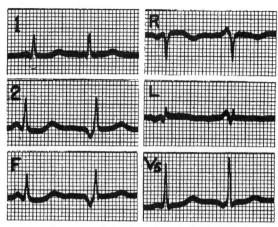

FIGURE 11–4 Junctional premature beats with antecedent P′ waves. In each lead the first beat is a sinus beat, and the second is a junctional premature beat with a short PR interval and typical P wave polarity. (From Marriott JLH. Practical Electrocardiography, 8th ed. Baltimore: Williams & Wilkins, 1988, p 154.)

JUNCTIONAL OR NODAL PREMATURE BEATS (JPBs)

ECG Diagnostic Points

- Junctional P waves may activate the atria retrogradely, and the retrograde P wave may precede the QRS complex (Fig. 11–4). Retrograde conduction may not be observed, and the P wave becomes lost in the QRS complex (Fig. 11–5). Occasionally the P wave follows the QRS complex.
- The P wave when visible is inverted in leads II, III, aVF, V_1, V_5, and V_6 and is upright in leads I, aVR, and aVL.
- The P wave may precede the QRS complex by ≤ 0.11 second.
- The term *upper nodal* or *mid* or *lower nodal rhythm* has been replaced by the term *junctional rhythm.*

VENTRICULAR PREMATURE BEATS (VPBs)

ECG Diagnostic Points

- Wide, bizarre, premature QRST complex, with ST segment sloping off in the direction opposite to the abnormal QRS complex (Figs. 11–6 to 11–8).
- No preceding premature P waves. Retrograde conduction of ectopic ventricular impulses occurs often; the retrograde P wave is usually hidden in the ventricular complex but occasionally can cause retrograde capture of the atria, and the inverted P wave may be observed following the VPB (Fig. 11–7).
- A VPB is followed usually by a fully compensatory pause, but this rule is often broken, and pauses may be less than compensatory.
- VPB duration generally is ≥ 0.11 second, but occasionally VPBs can be as short as 0.1 second in duration.

Text continued on page 206

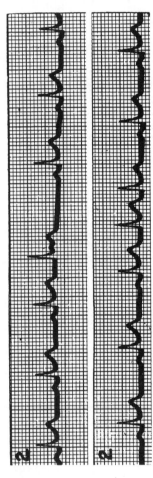

FIGURE 11–5 Junctional premature beats without retrograde conduction. In the upper strip the fourth beat is a junctional extrasystole. In the lower strip the fourth and fifth beats are a pair of junctional premature beats. In neither strip is the regular sinus discharge interrupted by retrograde conduction. (From Marriott JLH. Practical Electrocardiography, 8th ed. Baltimore: Williams & Wilkins, 1988, p 154.)

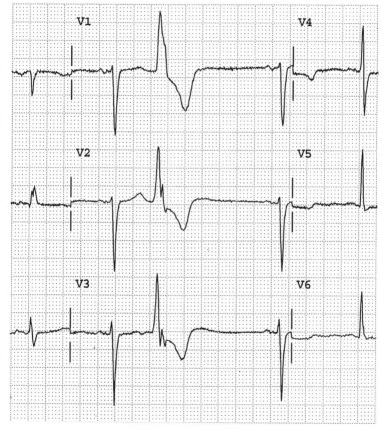

FIGURE 11–6   A ventricular premature beat: the ST segment slopes in the direction opposite to the slope of the abnormal QRS complex; V₁ shows a left "rabbit ear" larger than the right "rabbit ear."

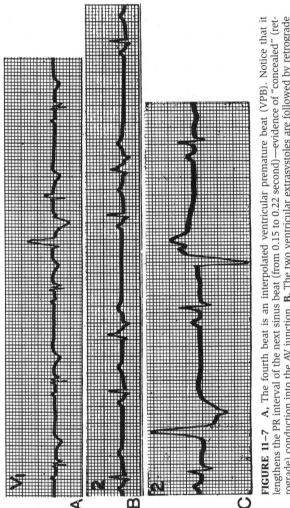

FIGURE 11–7 A, The fourth beat is an interpolated ventricular premature beat (VPB). Notice that it lengthens the PR interval of the next sinus beat (from 0.15 to 0.22 second)—evidence of "concealed" (retrograde) conduction into the AV junction. **B,** The two ventricular extrasystoles are followed by retrograde (inverted) P waves at normal RP' intervals of 0.17 and 0.19 second. **C,** Both VPBs are followed by retrograde P waves at abnormally prolonged RP' intervals (0.28 and 0.22 second). (From Marriott JLH. Practical Electrocardiography, 8th ed. Baltimore: Williams & Wilkins, 1988, p 145.)

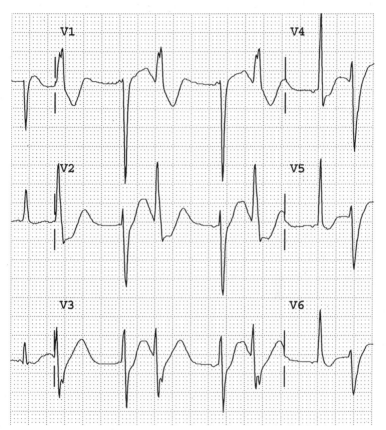

FIGURE 11–8 Ventricular bigeminy.

- If in V₁ the abnormal looking QRS shows a left "rabbit ear" larger than the right "rabbit ear" (Fig. 11-6), a diagnosis of VPB is certain. If the left "rabbit ear" is smaller than the right, no firm conclusion can be made from the morphology alone.
- Figure 11-8*A* shows ventricular bigeminy.
- A run of two beats is called a couplet; of three consecutive beats, a triplet or a salvo of three (Fig. 11-9); more than three consecutive VPBs is called ventricular tachycardia (VT) (Fig. 11-10).

With multifocal VPBs the coupling intervals vary; with unifocal VPBs the coupling intervals are equal. Unifocal VPBs are of little consequence. VPBs that occur early, close to the T wave or R on T, and that are multifocal or multiform, occurring as couplets or triplets, may trigger VT (Fig. 11-11).

VPBs occur commonly in normal and abnormal hearts. The word *beat* denotes an electrical and mechanical event and is preferred to the word *contraction*, which implies a mechanical event. The text uses the terms *VPBs* and *APBs*, not *VPCs* and *APCs*.

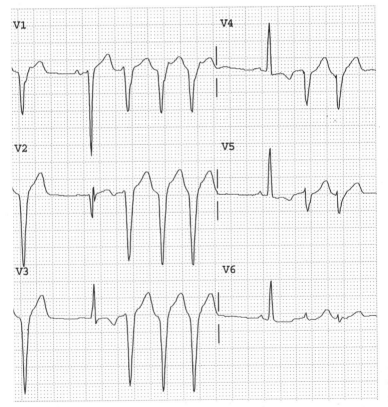

FIGURE 11-9 Ventricular premature beats occur in pairs (couplets) and in salvos of three (triplets).

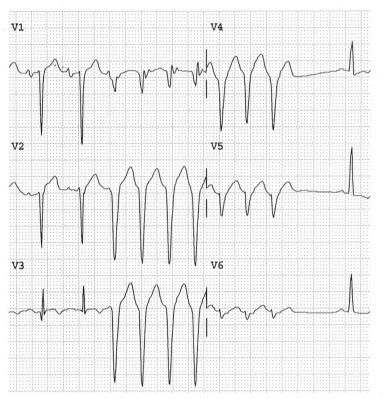

FIGURE 11–10   Short run of nonsustained ventricular tachycardia.

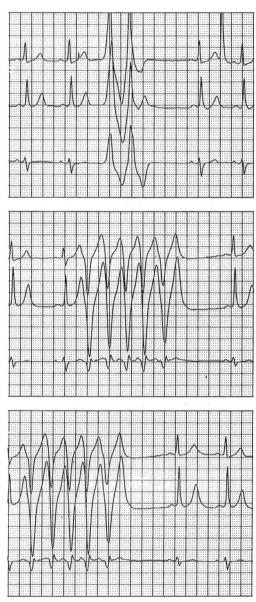

FIGURE 11-11 Holter monitor showing multifocal ventricular premature beats: couplet, salvo, nonsustained ventricular tachycardia. (From Khan MG. On Call Cardiology. Philadelphia: WB Saunders, 1997, p 119.)

BRADYARRHYTHMIAS

FIRST-DEGREE AV BLOCK

ECG Diagnostic Points
- PR interval > 0.2 second, usually 0.22 to 0.48 second but can be as long as 0.8 second (Fig. 11–12); some normal individuals have intervals up to 0.22 second.
- The PR interval should be constant.
- Each P wave should be followed by a QRS complex.

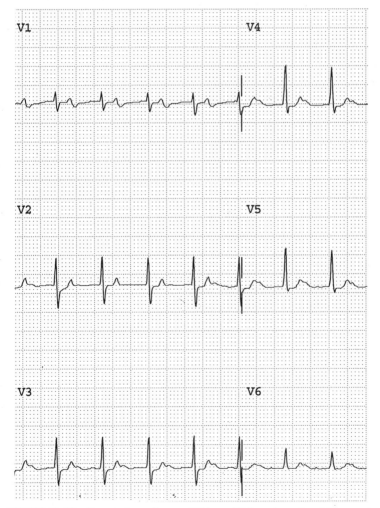

FIGURE 11–12   Sinus tachycardia: rate 118 bpm; PR is prolonged to 0.28 second: first-degree AV block.

SECOND-DEGREE AV BLOCK: MOBITZ TYPE I (WENCKEBACH)

ECG Diagnostic Criteria
- Progressive prolongation of the PR interval until the P wave is blocked, the impulse fails to conduct to the ventricles, and the QRS beat is dropped.
- Following the dropped QRS beat the PR interval reverts to near normal; the PR interval that follows the blocked P wave is always short.
- The RR interval containing the nonconducted P wave is shorter than two of the shorter cycles, i.e., shorter than the sum of two PP intervals (Fig. 11–13).
- Because there is usually a progressive shortening of the RR interval before a P wave is blocked, beats often are grouped in pairs (bigeminy) or trios (trigeminy). This group pattern is a hallmark of Wenckebach but is not necessary for the diagnosis (Fig. 11–14).

SECOND-DEGREE AV BLOCK: MOBITZ TYPE II

ECG Diagnostic Criteria
- At least two regular and consecutive atrial impulses are conducted with the same PR interval before the dropped beat (Fig. 11–15).
- With type 2, high grade second-degree AV block (Fig. 11–15*B*), two or more than two consecutive atrial impulses fail to be conducted because of the block itself. The diagnosis is strengthened if the atrial rate is slow (< 135 beats per minute [bpm]) in the absence of interference by an escaping subsidiary pacemaker that may prevent conduction.
- Intermittent nonconducted P waves are observed but with no evidence for atrial prematurity.
- The RR interval containing the nonconducted P wave is equal to two PP intervals.
- The PR interval remains constant and is normal or slightly prolonged.
- The ventricular rhythm is irregular because of nonconducted beats.
- If the conduction problem is in the His bundle, the QRS complex remains narrow, but it will be > 0.12 second if the lesion is below the His bundle.

COMPLETE (THIRD-DEGREE) AV BLOCK

ECG Diagnostic Criteria
- P waves are sinus and plentiful with few QRS complexes.
- AV dissociation: no relationship between P waves and QRS complexes: complete absence of AV conduction (Figs. 11–16 and 11–17). Note that AV dissociation may occur in the absence of third-degree AV block; the clue here is that the ventricular rate is faster than the atrial rate.
- The RR intervals are regular. The QRS complex is narrow if the site of block is in the AV node with an escape rhythm originating in the AV junction. the QRS is wide if the escaped rhythm originates from the ventricle or in the AV junction in the presence of bundle branch block.

Text continued on page 216

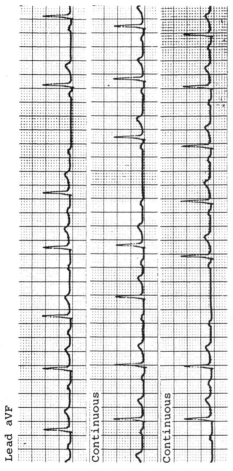

Lead aVF

Continuous

Continuous

FIGURE 11-13 Type I second-degree AV block without the typical Wenckebach phenomenon. Note the random variation of the PR and RR intervals except that the PR interval that follows the blocked P waves is always short. The QRS complexes that terminate the pauses may be junctional escape beats. (From Chou TC. Electrocardiography in Clinical Practice, 4th ed. Philadelphia: WB Saunders, 1996, p 452.)

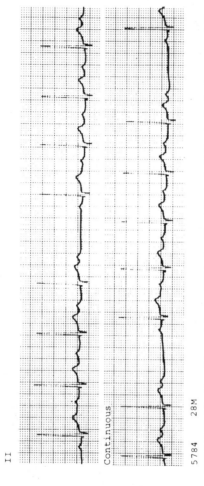

FIGURE 11–14   Type I second-degree AV block without the typical Wenckenbach phenomenon. There is no progressive shortening of the RR interval before the block. (From Chou TC. Electrocardiography in Clinical Practice, 4th ed. Philadelphia: WB Saunders, 1996, p 452.)

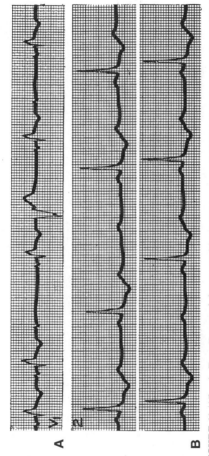

FIGURE 11–15 **A,** Type II second-degree AV block. Two consecutive PR intervals are unchanged before the dropped beat. The conducted beats have a normal PR interval and show RBBB; the fourth beat is a right ventricular premature beat. **B,** High-grade second-degree AV block. Sinus rhythm with 2:1 and 3:1 AV block. (From Marriott JLH. Practical Electrocardiography, 8th ed. Baltimore: Williams & Wilkins, 1988, p 370.)

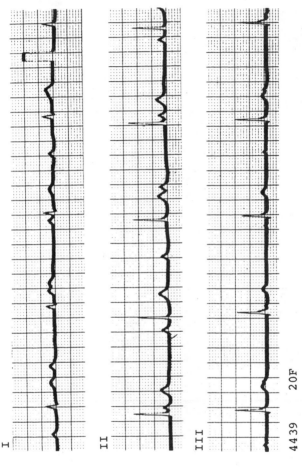

4439   20F

FIGURE 11–16 Congenital complete AV block. The narrow QRS complexes suggest that the escape pacemaker is junctional in origin. (From Chou TC. Electrocardiography in Clinical Practice, 4th ed. Philadelphia: WB Saunders, 1996, p 457.)

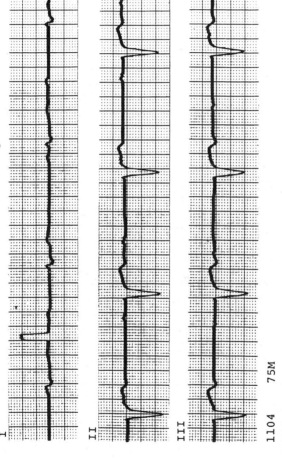

I

II

III

1104   75M

FIGURE 11–17 Complete AV block with idioventricular rhythm. The QRS complexes are abnormally wide and are different from those seen during sinus rhythm. The ventricular rate is 36 bpm. (From Chou TC. Electrocardiography in Clinical Practice, 4th ed. Philadelphia: WB Saunders, 1996, p 457.)

- The atrial rate is faster than the ventricular rate.
- Ventricular rate usually is very slow, < 45 bpm, but with congenital AV block, rates may be 40 to 60 bpm (Fig. 11–16).
- With complete AV block, anterograde conduction never occurs, but in less than 20% of complete AV blocks, retrograde conduction to the atria occurs.

Note that AV dissociation may occur in the absence of third-degree AV block.

TACHYCARDIAS

Differentiate tachycardias as narrow QRS or wide QRS, then into regular or irregular (Fig. 11–18).

NARROW QRS TACHYCARDIA

A comparison of the entire 12-lead ECG during tachycardia with the ECG in sinus rhythm is most helpful for clarifying the diagnosis. Careful assessment of leads II, III, aVF, V_1, and V_6 should reveal clues to the diagnosis.

Sinus Tachycardia

Always consider sinus tachycardia if the rate is 100 to 140 bpm because it is the most common cause of narrow QRS tachycardia (Fig. 11–19). With faster rates the sinus P wave may be hidden in the T waves and mimic supraventricular tachycardia (SVT) or atrial flutter. The sinus P wave can be revealed by carotid massage.

Atrioventricular Nodal Reentrant Tachycardia (AVNRT)

AVNRT is the most common cause of a paroxysmal narrow, regular QRS tachycardia. The ventricles are activated from the anterograde path of the circuit, with activation of the atrium by the retrograde path (Fig. 11–20).

ECG Diagnostic Points
- A rapid, regular rhythm, usually 150 to 225 bpm is present; a rate of > 230 bpm should prompt the search for Wolff-Parkinson-White (WPW) syndrome.
- A QRS of < 0.12 second.
- In more than 50% of cases, P waves are hidden within the QRS complex and are not visible; the QRS complex is identical to that of a tracing during sinus rhythm (Fig. 11–20).
- In approximately 45% of cases, P waves appear hidden, but on careful scrutiny they are visible at the end of the QRS in leads II, III, and aVF as they distort the terminal forces of the QRS complex, resulting in pseudo-S waves in leads II, III, and aVF (Fig. 11–21). The distortion causes a pseudo r′ wave in lead V_1 that mimics RSr′ or incomplete right bundle branch block (RBBB) (Figs. 11–20, 11–21B, and 11–22).
- In less than 5% of cases, P waves are discernible at the beginning of the QRS and cause pseudo-q waves in leads II, III, and aVF.

Text continued on page 221

STEP 11

A   **Narrow QRS tachycardia**

Regular

Sinus tachycardia

Atrioventricular nodal reentrant
tachycardia (AVNRT)

Atrial flutter (with fixed AV
conduction)

Atrial tachycardia (paroxysmal
and nonparoxysmal)

WPW syndrome (orthodromic
circus movement tachycardia)

Irregular

Atrial fibrillation

Atrial flutter (with variable AV
conduction)

Atrial tachycardia (variable AV
block or Wenckebach)

Multifocal atrial tachycardia

B   **Wide QRS tachycardia**

Regular

Ventricular tachycardia

Supraventricular tachycardia
(with preexisting or functional
bundle branch block)

   Atrioventricular nodal reentrant
     tachycardia
   WPW syndrome (orthodromic)
   Sinus tachycardia
   Atrial tachycardia
   Atrial flutter with fixed AV
     conduction

WPW syndrome (antidromic,
preexcited tachycardia)

Irregular

Atrial fibrillation (with bundle
branch block or with WPW
syndrome [antidromic])

Atrial flutter (varying AV
conduction, with bundle branch
block or WPW syndrome
[antidromic])

Torsades de pointes

FIGURE 11–18   Method for rapid ECG interpretation. **A,** Step 11: The differential
diagnosis of narrow QRS tachycardia. **B,** Step 11: The differential diagnosis of wide
QRS tachycardia. (Modified from Khan MG. Heart Disease Diagnosis & Therapy. Baltimore: Williams & Wilkins, 1996, p 273.)

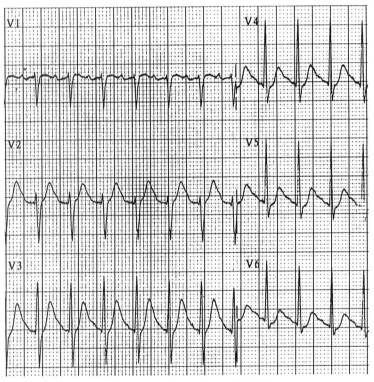

FIGURE 11–19 Sinus tachycardia 165 bpm.

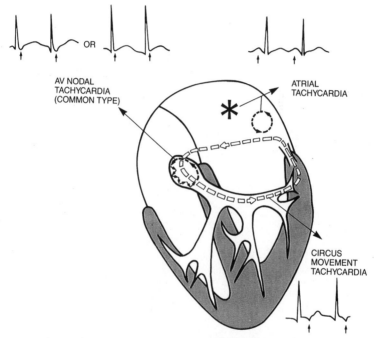

FIGURE 11–20 A representation of the sites of origin and mechanism of paroxysmal supraventricular tachycardia (SVT) as determined by the position and polarity of the P waves in relation to the QRS complexes. In atrial tachycardia the P wave precedes the QRS; its polarity in lead III depends on its location. In AV nodal reentry tachycardia the P wave is buried within the QRS or may distort the end of the QRS; that portion of the QRS is then negative in lead III. In circus movement tachycardia the P wave follows the QRS. (From Wellens JJH, Conover MB. The ECG in Emergency Decision Making. Philadelphia: WB Saunders, 1992, p 75.)

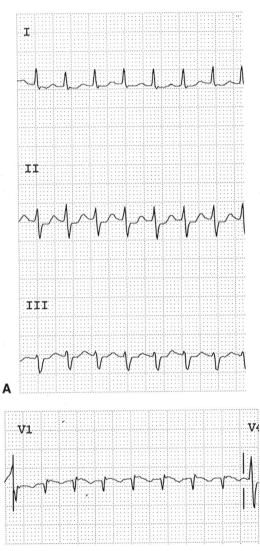

FIGURE 11–21 **A,** The limb leads of a patient with supraventricular tachycardia: rate 184 bpm. Note the distortion of the terminal QRS in lead III, a pseudo-S wave: typical features of the common form of AV nodal reentrant tachycardia (AVNRT). **B,** The V_1 lead in the same patient. Note the distortion of the terminal QRS resulting in a pseudo-R': typical feature of the common form of AVNRT.

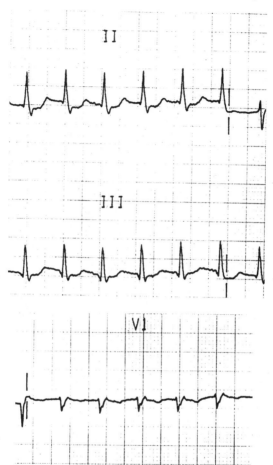

FIGURE 11–22   AV nodal reentrant tachycardia (AVNRT): rate 140 bpm. Note pseudo-R′ wave in V₁, typical of the common type of AVNRT.

- In a rare form of AVNRT, P waves are negative in leads II, III, and aVF but follow the QRS after a prolonged duration such that the RP interval is ≥ the PR interval. It is impossible to distinguish this rare form of AVNRT from the rare-type WPW circus movement tachycardia using the retrograde, slow accessory pathway to activate the atria (see WPW Syndrome).

Paroxysmal Atrial Tachycardia (PAT) with or without AV Block

ECG Diagnostic Points

- The P wave precedes the QRS, and its contour is different from that of the sinus P wave. P waves are often small, are not easily identified, and may be hidden in the T wave or QRS; the arrhythmia may be mistaken for sinus tachycardia or AV junctional tachycardia. The PR interval is normal or prolonged.

- The morphology of the P waves depends on the location of the ectopic atrial pacemaker (Fig. 11–23). The RR intervals are equal except for a warm-up period in the automatic type.
- The atrial rate may range from 110 to 260 bpm. If the atrial rate is not rapid and AV conduction is not depressed, each P wave may conduct to the ventricle. With digitalis excess, AV conduction may be delayed, resulting in PAT with block, but digitalis toxicity is not the only cause of this arrhythmia (Fig. 11–24).
- Variable AV conduction occurs: A 2:1 conduction is common; a 3:1 conduction or Wenckebach's phenomenon may occur, causing an irregular rhythm (Fig. 11–25). At times the varying AV block may result in an irregular ventricular rhythm that may be mistaken for atrial fibrillation.

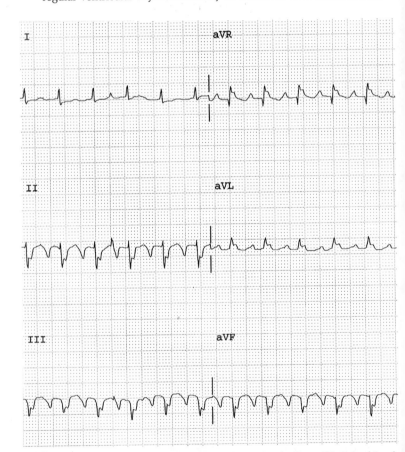

FIGURE 11–23 Atrial tachycardia. The P waves are barely discernible in lead I and are inverted in II, III, and aVF. There is 2:1 AV block. The atrial rate is 264 bpm; ventricular rate 132 bpm. Note the isoelectric baseline between the P wave and the QRS complex.

Lead II

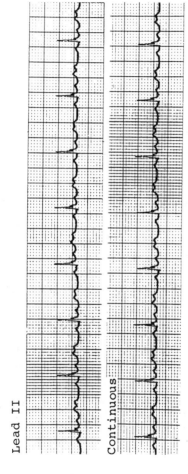

Continuous

FIGURE 11–24 Paroxysmal atrial tachycardia with block. There is 3:1 AV conduction. The patient was not receiving digitalis. (From Chou TC. Electrocardiography in Clinical Practice, 4th ed. Philadelphia: WB Saunders, 1996, p 350.)

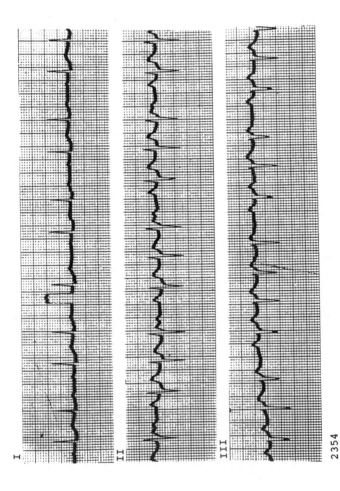

2 3 5 4

FIGURE 11–25   Paroxysmal atrial tachycardia with block. A Wenckebach phenomenon is present. There is a gradual lengthening of the PR interval and shortening of the RR interval before the block occurs; therefore irregular. (From Chou TC. Electrocardiography in Clinical Practice, 4th ed. Philadelphia: WB Saunders, 1996, p 351.)

- An isoelectric baseline exists between the P wave and the QRS complex (Figs. 11–23 to 11–25).
- The differentiation of atrial tachycardia and atrial flutter may be difficult if the atrial rate is rapid; carotid sinus massage or adenosine brings out the flutter waves if atrial flutter is present.
- Atrial tachycardia persists despite the development of AV block, and this feature excludes WPW syndrome.

Persistent ("Incessant") Atrial Tachycardia

The incessant nature of this rare tachycardia may cause dilated (congestive) cardiomyopathy.

ECG Diagnostic Points
- The rhythm is regular.
- The P wave precedes the QRS complex. The P wave polarity depends on the site of origin in the atrium.
- Variable AV conduction of 1:1 and 2:1, including Wenckebach's phenomenon.
- Carotid sinus massage or adenosine increases AV block and facilitates the diagnosis.

Multifocal Atrial Tachycardia (Chaotic Atrial Tachycardia)

ECG Diagnostic Points
- An atrial rate of 100 to 140 bpm.
- Frequent multifocal premature beats. At least three different P wave morphologies with changing PR intervals in one lead (Fig. 11–26); isoelectric baseline between P waves.
- The rhythm is completely irregular; variable PR, RR, and RP intervals.
- The absence of one dominant atrial pacemaker such as sinus rhythm with multifocal APBs.
- Causes include chronic obstructive pulmonary disease (COPD), theophylline, and digitalis (rarely).

Wolff-Parkinson-White (WPW) Syndrome

ECG Diagnostic Criteria
- QRS complex duration of ≥ 0.11 second; in approximately 20% of individuals the QRS complex may not be > 0.1 second. PR < 0.12 second.
- A delta wave is prominent, often in V_3 through V_6, and is a subtle finding in some leads (Fig. 11–27).
- In type A WPW syndrome a tall R wave present in V_1 and V_2 can mimic right ventricular hypertrophy (RVH), RBBB, or posterior infarction (Fig. 11–27 and Table 1–3, p. 17).
- In type B WPW pattern the QRS complex is predominantly negative in V_1 through V_3 and upright in V_5 and V_6; the pattern resembles left bundle branch block (LBBB) (Fig. 11–28).
- Possible mimicry of inferior myocardial infarction (MI) (Figs. 11–27 and 11–29).

Text continued on page 230

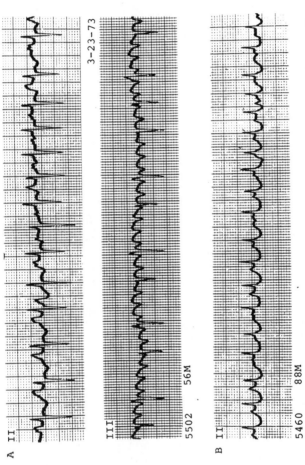

A II

III

5502   56M

B II

5460   88M

FIGURE 11–26   Multifocal atrial tachycardia. **A,** The patient has chronic obstructive pulmonary disease (COPD). The tracing on 3-14-73 shows multifocal atrial tachycardia. The rhythm changes to atrial flutter with varying AV conduction on 3-23-73. **B,** Tracing obtained from an 88-year-old man with mitral insufficiency. The multifocal atrial tachycardia closely resembles atrial fibrillation with rapid ventricular response. (From Chou TC. Electrocardiography in Clinical Practice, 4th ed. Philadelphia: WB Saunders, 1996, p 353.)

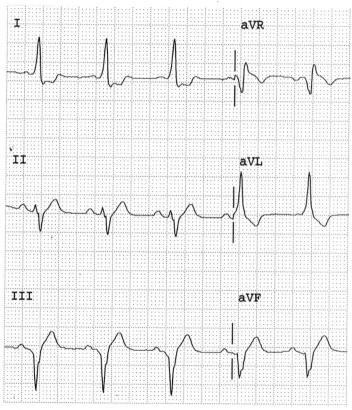

A

FIGURE 11–27   Features of WPW syndrome. Prominent delta waves in V_2 through V_5 and very short PR interval. Note how this mimics inferior infarction.

Figure continued on following page

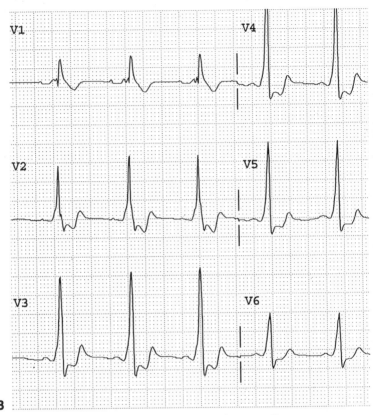

B

FIGURE 11–27 *Continued* See legend on preceding page.

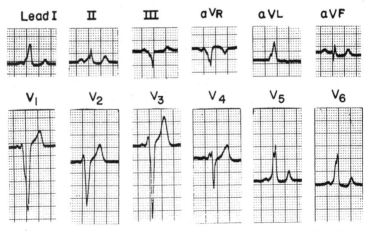

FIGURE 11–28 Type B WPW pattern in a 35-year-old healthy man. The tracing resembles closely that of complete left bundle branch block. (From Chou TC. Electrocardiography in Clinical Practice, 4th ed. Philadelphia: WB Saunders, 1996, p 477.)

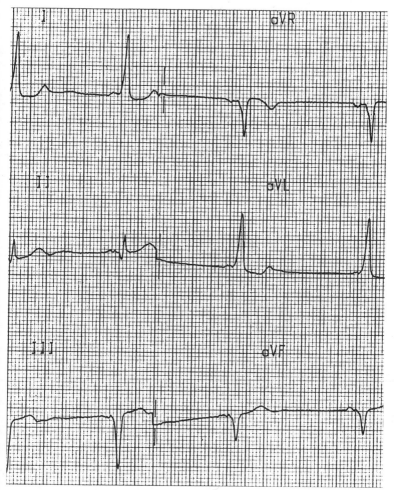

FIGURE 11–29 Limb leads in patient with WPW syndrome mimic inferior infarction.

Clues during Tachycardia

- Narrow QRS complex tachycardia, regular rhythm.
- P waves follow the QRS at a distance; shape depends on the location of the accessory pathway. With a left lateral accessory pathway the P wave is negative in lead I; if the location is posteroseptal, P waves are negative in leads II, III, and aVF and positive in aVR and aVL.
- In the common orthodromic circus movement tachycardia the RP interval is shorter than the PR interval because of retrograde use of the fast accessory pathway to activate the atria (Figs. 11–20 and 11–30).
- In a rare form of orthodromic circus movement tachycardia, with retrograde activation of the atria through a slow conducting accessory pathway, the P wave occurs late retrogradely; thus the RP interval is longer than or equal to the PR interval and the P wave is negative in leads II, III, aVF, and V_4 through V_6. This arrhythmia pattern is similar

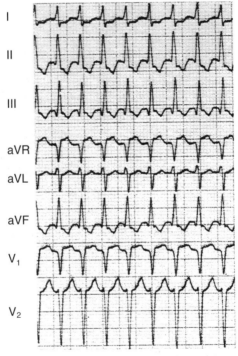

FIGURE 11–30   An example of a circus movement tachycardia using a concealed accessory pathway. The diagnosis is based on the position of the P wave during the tachycardia. Negative P waves are clearly visible in leads II, III, and aVF following the QRS complex. The P waves during the tachycardia are positive in leads aVR and aVL, indicating a posteroseptal atrial insertion of the accessory pathway. (From Wellens JJH, Conover MB. The ECG in Emergency Decision Making. Philadelphia: WB Saunders, 1992, p 86.)

to the rare form of AVNRT described earlier (Fig. 11–31). This rare type of WPW syndrome may manifest as a persistent (incessant) orthodromic circus movement tachycardia and cause a dilated cardiomyopathy with congestive heart failure.

- Electrical alternans sometimes occurs during orthodromic circus movement tachycardia but occurs rarely with other narrow QRS tachycardias (see Figs. 10–10 and 10–11).

Summary Differential Diagnosis of Narrow QRS Regular Tachycardia

- If AV block is present or can be produced by carotid sinus massage or adenosine, WPW syndrome can be ruled out; atrial flutter and atrial tachycardia persist despite AV block.

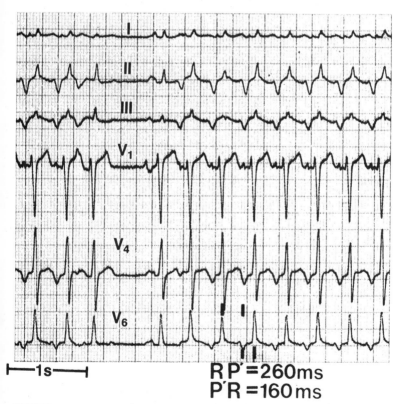

FIGURE 11–31 Incessant circus movement tachycardia using a slowly conducting concealed accessory pathway for retrograde conduction. The diagnosis is made because the patient is in tachycardia most of the time with an RP interval greater than the PR interval. The tachycardia is temporarily terminated by an atrial premature beat, which is conducted to the ventricle. There is a pause due to retrograde block in the accessory pathway. Then the sinus node escapes for one beat and the circus movement tachycardia begins again. (From Wellens JJH, Conover MB. The ECG in Emergency Decision Making. Philadelphia: WB Saunders, 1992, p 89.)

- If the P wave is hidden within the QRS or is distorting the terminal QRS, causing a pseudo-S in leads II, III, and AVF or a pseudo r′ in V₁, the diagnosis is the common form of AVNRT (Figs. 11–20 to 11–22).
- A negative P wave in lead I suggests WPW syndrome or left atrial tachycardia.
- A P wave following the QRS complex distinctly with an RP interval shorter than the PR interval is diagnostic of the most common type of WPW syndrome, orthodromic circus movement tachycardia (Fig. 11–30).
- An RP interval ≥ the PR interval indicates the rare WPW orthodromic type, the rare type of AVNRT, or atrial tachycardia (Fig. 11–31).
- Positive P waves in leads II, III, and aVF with atrial tachycardia rule out AVNRT or WPW syndrome tachycardia.
- P waves negative in leads II, III, and aVF suggest AVNRT or WPW syndrome.
- A ventricular rate > 220 bpm with QRS alternans usually indicates WPW syndrome.
- A ventricular rate > 250 bpm with RR intervals ≤ 240 ms (six small squares) suggests WPW syndrome.

Four Types of WPW Syndrome Tachycardia

A. The most common tachycardia is termed *orthodromic circus movement tachycardia:* activation of the ventricles via the AV node and His bundle; the impulse retrogradely uses the fast accessory tract to activate the atria; thus the P wave is close to the preceding QRS complex, and the RP interval is shorter than the PR interval.

B. *Rare orthodromic tachycardia.* Similar activation of the ventricle via the AV node and His bundle but return of the impulse to the atria via slow accessory tract; therefore the P wave follows the QRS at a distance, making the RP interval ≥ the PR interval. This arrhythmia mimics the rare form of AVNRT.

C. *Rare antidromic tachycardia.* Anterograde (preexcited tachycardia) use of bypass tract to activate the ventricle, causing tachycardia similar to VT or atrial flutter or fibrillation with a wide QRS complex (see discussion of wide QRS tachycardia).

D. *Rare antidromic anterograde conduction* using two or more accessory pathways, resulting in wide QRS tachycardia.

Diagnosis Based on Carotid Sinus Massage or IV Adenosine

- AVNRT converts to sinus rhythm or no effect.
- Circus movement tachycardia reverts to sinus rhythm or no effect.
- Persistent atrial tachycardia: increased AV block facilitates recognition of the atrial origin, temporary slowing of heart rate with AV block, or no effect.
- Atrial flutter: temporary slowing of the ventricular rate reveals flutter waves if not previously visible or no effect.

Atrial Flutter

- A sawtooth pattern in leads II, III, and aVF (Fig. 11–32). The downward deflection of the F waves has a gradual slope followed by an abrupt up-

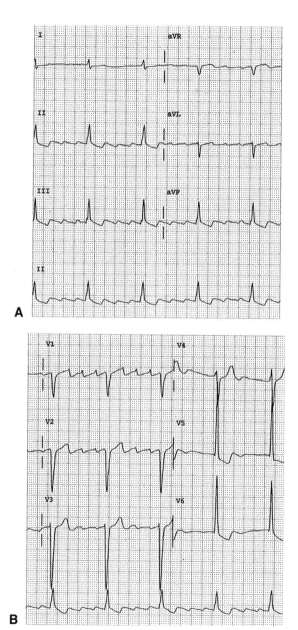

FIGURE 11–32   Atrial flutter. (From Khan MG. On Call Cardiology. Philadelphia: WB Saunders, 1997, p 133.)

ward deflection; this results in the typical sharp spikes of the sawtooth pattern: Positive "spiky" P-like waves in lead V_1; negative P-like waves in leads V_5 and V_6; and nearly no atrial activity in lead I; occasionally leads V_5 and V_6 may show negligible atrial activity (Fig. 11–32).

- A ventricular response of 150 bpm is typical of atrial flutter. The atrial rate is often 300 bpm. With 2:1 AV conduction the ventricular response is 150 bpm. This 2:1 ratio may not be apparent because an F wave may be partially obscured by the QRS complex and the second F wave is hidden in the T wave (Fig. 11–33). This pattern mimics sinus tachycardia or reentrant junctional tachycardia. Carotid sinus massage should reveal sinus P waves or F waves. Conduction ratios of 2:1 and 4:1 may occur. The ventricular rate may vary from 100 to 230 bpm. A ventricular response of > 250 bpm suggests WPW syndrome.
- The rhythm is regular but becomes irregular when there is variable AV conduction.
- The atrial rate varies from 250 to 400 bpm but can be < 200 bpm in patients taking quinidine.

Atrial Fibrillation

ECG Diagnostic Points
- RR intervals are completely irregular (irregularly irregular) (Fig. 11–34).
- Irregular undulation of the baseline is usually most prominent in V_1; these may be gross (Fig. 11–35) or barely perceptible, described as coarse and fine fibrillation, respectively. Occasionally there may be no recognizable undulations of the baseline, and careful measurement of the RR interval is necessary to detect slight irregularities.
- The atrial rate ranges from 400 to 700 bpm; there is variable AV conduction, resulting in a chaotic ventricular response.
- QRS complexes often vary in amplitude.
- The heart rate is commonly 100 to 180 bpm but can accelerate to > 200 bpm. Rates of > 210 bpm with the QRS complex $\geq$ 0.12 second should suggest WPW syndrome. With WPW antidromic tachycardia, wide QRS tachycardia with rates of 250 to 320 bpm may occur.

WIDE QRS TACHYCARDIA

ECG Diagnostic Steps
- Define the QRS duration $\geq$ 0.12 second.
- Define the tachycardia as regular or irregular (Fig. 11–18*B*).

Regular Wide QRS Tachycardia

- Ventricular tachycardia. Consider all wide QRS regular tachycardias VT until proven otherwise.
- SVT with preexisting or functional bundle branch block: these include AVNRT, orthodromic circus movement tachycardia (WPW), atrial tachycardia, and atrial flutter with fixed AV conduction.
- Antidromic circus movement tachycardia, preexcited tachycardia (WPW).

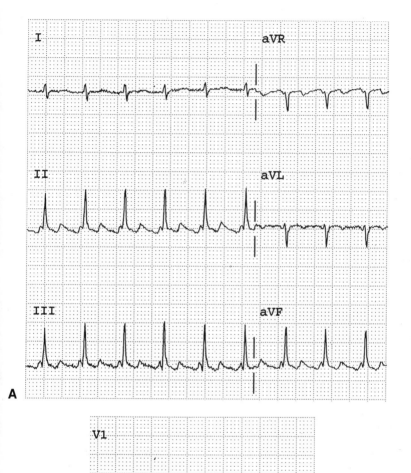

FIGURE 11–33   Atrial flutter: atrial rate 270 bpm; ventricular rate 135 bpm. Note the downward deflection of F waves in leads II, III, and aVF has a gradual slope followed by an abrupt upward deflection. This causes the sawtooth pattern. Alternate F waves coincide with the QRS complex, and the diagnosis may be missed.

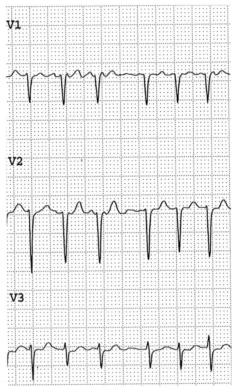

A

FIGURE 11–34 Atrial fibrillation with a rapid ventricular response of 174 bpm.

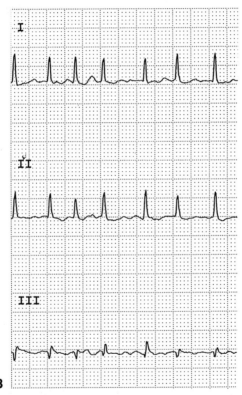

B

FIGURE 11–34 *Continued*   See legend on opposite page.

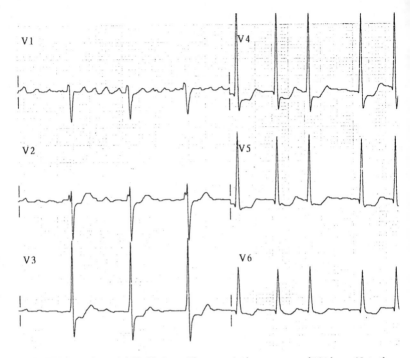

FIGURE 11–35 Atrial fibrillation with a ventricular response of 104 bpm. Note the coarse atrial fibrillation in V_1.

Ventricular Tachycardia

The ECG diagnosis of VT requires the assessment of all 12 ECG leads. The diagnosis of VT can be confidently made by a careful scrutiny of the morphologic pattern of the QRS complexes in V_1 through V_6.

- If the QRS complexes are all negative in V_1 through V_6, i.e., negative precordial concordance, the diagnosis of VT is certain; also, predominantly QRS complexes in V_4 through V_6 are diagnostic of VT (Figs. 11–36 to 11–38).
- The presence of a QR complex in one or more of precordial leads V_2 through V_6 is diagnostic (Fig. 11–36). Note that negative precordial concordance is diagnostic of VT but that positive concordance (all complexes positive in V_1 through V_6) can be due to VT or circus movement antidromic tachycardia WPW syndrome (Fig. 11–37).
- The RS interval should be > 0.1 second, measured from the R wave to the nadir of the S wave in any precordial lead.
- AV dissociation: the presence of more QRS complexes than P waves support the diagnosis of VT, but P wave identification may be difficult. The terminal portion of the T wave or initial parts of the QRS may resemble P waves, leading to an incorrect diagnosis of SVT. Also, in some cases of VT, 1:1 VA conduction may be observed because retrograde impulse conduction to the atria from the ventricular focus often occurs. Thus, AV dissociation is not a reliable diagnostic point.

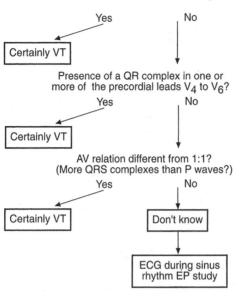

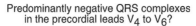

Predominantly negative QRS complexes
in the precordial leads V_4 to V_6?

Yes — Certainly VT

No →

Presence of a QR complex in one or
more of the precordial leads V_4 to V_6?

Yes — Certainly VT

No →

AV relation different from 1:1?
(More QRS complexes than P waves?)

Yes — Certainly VT

No → Don't know

ECG during sinus
rhythm EP study

FIGURE 11–36 Differential diagnosis of wide QRS complex tachycardia as it should be used in clinical practice. *VT,* ventricular tachycardia. (From Steurer G, Gursoy S, Frey B, et al. Clin Cardiol 1994;17:308. Copyrighted and reprinted with the permission of Clinical Cardiology Publishing Company, Inc., and/or the Foundation for Advances in Medicine and Science, Inc., Mahwah, NJ 07430-0832, USA.)

- The presence of a QS or rS in V_6 or a net negative QRS in V_5, i.e., an r with a deep S in lead V_6, is typical of VT (Fig. 11–39).
- The morphology in V_1 may be helpful: if the left "rabbit ear" is taller than the right in lead V_1, VT is the most likely diagnosis (Figs. 11–37 and 11–39). Note that the rabbit ear may be subtle.
- With VT the axis is commonly –90° to ±180°. The axis may, however, be normal in patients with idiopathic VT and other varieties of VT.
- Positive concordance: positive QRS complex in V_1 through V_6 is suggestive of VT, but this pattern can be seen with WPW syndrome (Fig. 11–40). Negative precordial concordance is diagnostic of VT because this pattern does not occur during antidromic circus movement tachycardia (WPW syndrome) in which conduction is anterograde over the bypass tract.

Irregular Wide QRS Tachycardia

- Atrial fibrillation with bundle branch block or with the antidromic variety of WPW, anterograde conduction over the bypass tract (Fig. 11–41).
- Atrial flutter with varying AV conduction and bundle branch block or atrial flutter and varying AV conduction in the WPW syndrome with anterograde conduction (antidromic) over the bypass tract (Fig. 11–42).

Text continued on page 246

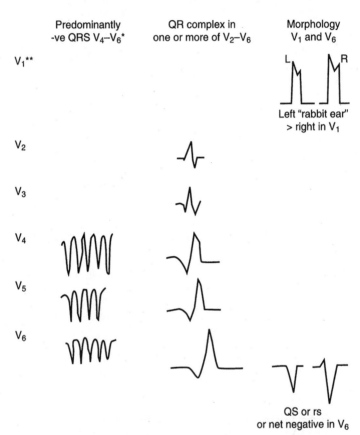

Predominantly -ve QRS V_4–V_6*	QR complex in one or more of V_2–V_6	Morphology V_1 and V_6
V_1**		Left "rabbit ear" > right in V_1

* = or concordant negativity in leads V_1 through V_4. Positive concordance in leads V_1 through V_6 can be caused by VT or Wolff-Parkinson-White anti-dromic (preexcited) tachycardia.

** = it is necessary to study the entire 12-lead tracing with particular emphasis on leads V_1 through V_6; lead II may be useful for assessment of P waves and AV dissociation.

FIGURE 11–37 Electrocardiographic hallmarks of ventricular tachycardia (VT). (From Khan MG. On Call Cardiology. Philadelphia, WB Saunders, 1997, p 142.)

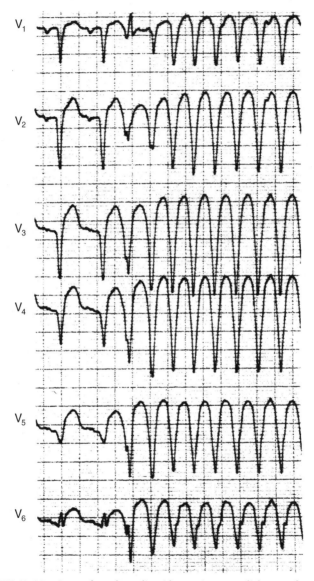

FIGURE 11–38   Onset of a tachycardia with negative precordial concordance. Negative precordial concordance indicates ventricular tachycardia, since such a pattern does not occur during anterograde conduction over an accessory pathway. (From Wellens JJH, Conover MB. The ECG in Emergency Decision Making. Philadelphia: WB Saunders, 1992, p 60.)

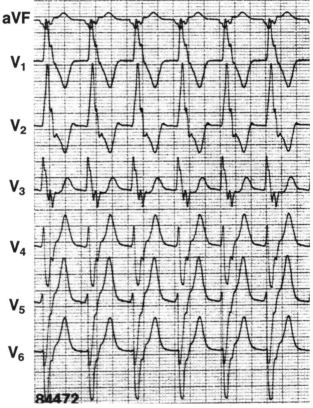

FIGURE 11–39 Ventricular tachycardia. Note the monophasic R wave in lead V_1 and the deep S in lead V_6, signs of ventricular tachycardia. The northwest axis is also a helpful clue. (From Wellens JJH, Conover MB. The ECG in Emergency Decision Making. Philadelphia: WB Saunders, 1992, p 51.)

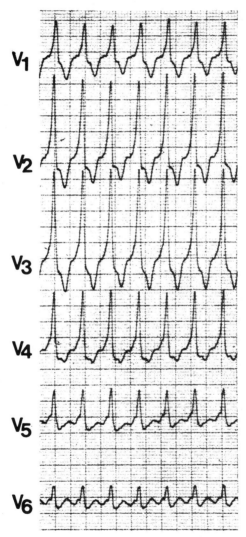

FIGURE 11–40   Broad QRS tachycardia with positive precordial concordance. The mechanism is atrial flutter with 2:1 conduction over a left-sided accessory pathway. (From Wellens JJH, Conover MB. The ECG in Emergency Decision Making. Philadelphia: WB Saunders, 1992, p 61.)

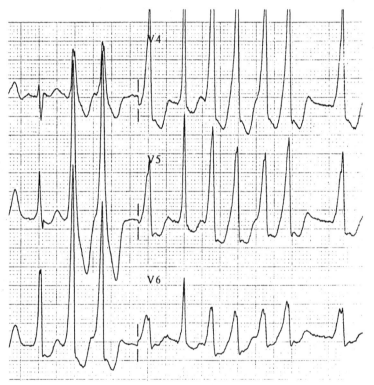

FIGURE 11–41 Atrial fibrillation with wide QRS tachycardia in a patient with Wolff-Parkinson-White syndrome: antidromic tachycardia.

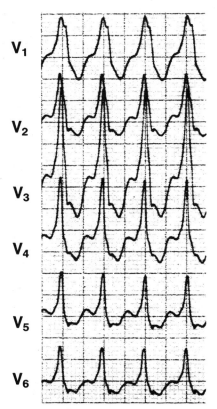

FIGURE 11–42 A 12-lead ECG from a patient with antidromic circus movement tachycardia. (From Wellens JJH, Conover MB. The ECG in Emergency Decision Making. Philadelphia: WB Saunders, 1992, p 67.)

- Torsades de pointes
  - Torsades is a polymorphic VT that usually occurs in the presence of a prolonged QT interval.
  - The RR interval is irregular; the QRS complexes show a typical twisting of the points.
  - The amplitudes of the complexes vary and appear alternately above and below the baseline (Fig. 11–43).

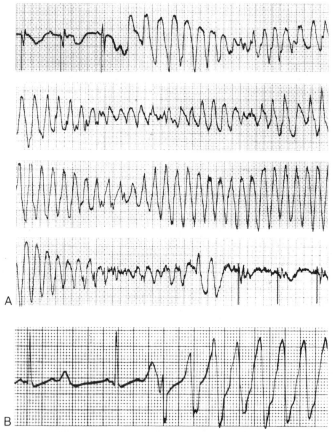

FIGURE 11–43 Torsades de pointes. **A,** Continuous recording monitor lead. A demand ventricular pacemaker (VVI) has been implanted because of type II second-degree AV block. After treatment with amiodarone for recurrent ventricular tachycardia (VT), the QT interval became prolonged (about 640 ms during paced beats), and the patient developed episodes of torsades de pointes. In this recording the tachycardia spontaneously terminates, and a paced ventricular rhythm is restored. Motion artifact is noted at the end of the recording as the patient lost consciousness. **B,** Tracing from a young boy with a congenital long QT syndrome. The QTU interval in the sinus beats is at least 600 ms. Note TU wave alternans in the first and second complexes. A late premature complex occurring in the downslope of the TU wave initiates an episode of VT. (From Braunwald E. Heart Disease: A Textbook of Cardiovascular Medicine, 5th ed. Philadelphia: WB Saunders, 1997, p 684.)

- The ventricular rate varies from 200 to 300 bpm but can reach 400 bpm and is usually not sustained, lasting 30 seconds to 1 minute.
- Longer episodes degenerate into ventricular fibrillation.
- Drugs and conditions that may precipitate torsades include the following:
  - Antiarrhythmics known to increase the QT interval: quinidine, procainamide, amiodarone, disopyramide, sotalol
  - Tricyclic antidepressants and phenothiazines
  - Histamine H_1 antagonists, such as astemizole and terfenadine
  - Antiviral and antifungal agents and antibiotics (see p. 176)
  - Hypokalemia, hypomagnesemia
  - Insecticide poisoning
  - Bradyarrhythmias
  - Congenital long QT syndrome
  - Subarachnoid hemorrhage
  - Chloroquine, pentamidine
  - Cocaine abuse

Index

Note: Page numbers in *italics* refer to illustrations; page numbers followed by t refer to tables.

A

Acquired immunodeficiency syndrome (AIDS), myocarditis in, vs. anteroseptal myocardial infarction, *126*

Adenosine, IV, in tachycardia, 232

Aneurysm, left ventricular, ST segment elevation in, *89, 90*

Antidromic anterograde conduction, 232. See also *Wolff-Parkinson-White syndrome.*

Antidromic tachycardia, 232, *244, 245.* See also *Wolff-Parkinson-White syndrome.*

Arrhythmias, 197–247. See also specific arrhythmias.
assessment of, *51, 52*

Atrial bigeminy, 197, *198, 199*

Atrial fibrillation, 234, *236–238*
digitalis toxicity and, *180*
with wide QRS tachycardia, 239, *244*

Atrial flutter, 232–234, *233, 235*

Atrial hypertrophy, 136–138
bilateral, *57, 137,* 138
left, 136–137
causes of, 136–137
diagnostic criteria for, 136, *137*
P wave in, 34, *35, 36,* 54, *57,* 58

Atrial hypertrophy *(Continued)*
right, 137–138
causes of, 138
diagnostic criteria for, 137–138, *138*
P wave in, 34, *35, 36,* 58

Atrial premature beats, 197–200
diagnosis of, 197, *198–200*
nonconduction of, 197, *200*
right bundle branch aberration and, *199*

Atrial septal defect, RSr′ variant in, *49, 69*

Atrial tachycardia, atrial premature beat and, 197, *199*
multifocal, 225, *226*
P wave in, 58
persistent, 225

Atrial trigeminy, *198*

Atrioventricular block, first-degree, 209, *209*
second-degree (Mobitz type I), 210, *211, 212*
second-degree (Mobitz type II), 210, *213*
third-degree (complete), 210, *214, 215,* 216

Atrioventricular junctional rhythm, P wave in, 54, *57*

Atrioventricular nodal reentrant tachycardia, 216, *219–221*, 232

B

Bifascicular block, *169*, *170–171*, 171
Bradyarrhythmias, 209–216, *209*, *211–215*
Bundle branch block, 64–73. See also *Left bundle branch block; Right bundle branch block.*
   atypical, 17, *17–19*

C

Cardiac tamponade, electrical alternans in, 183
Cardiomyopathy, hypertrophic, Q wave in, 63, *126–127*, 127
   ST segment elevation in, 90
Carotid sinus massage, in tachycardia, 232
Chaotic atrial tachycardia, 225, *226*
Cocaine abuse, in myocardial infarction, 109, *121*
   ST segment elevation in, 90
Cornell voltage criteria, for left ventricular hypertrophy, 141
Coronary artery spasm, ST segment elevation in, 90

D

Delta wave, in Wolff-Parkinson-White syndrome, 225, *227–228*
Depolarization, 59–63, *60*, *62*
Dextrocardia, with situs inversus, *50*, 179, *180*, *182*, 183
   without situs inversus, 183
Dextroposition, *182*, 183
Dextroversion, 183
Digitalis toxicity, 179, *180*

E

Einthoven's equilateral triangle, 160, *161*
Electrical alternans, 183, *184*
Electrical axis, 160–166, *161–163*, 163t
   assessment of, 43, *44–46*, 46t
   in ventricular tachycardia, 239
   left deviation of, 43, *44–46*, 46t, *162–163*, 163t, 164–165, *164*
   normal, 3t, *162–163*, 163t, 164
   right deviation of, 43, *44–45*, 46t, *162–163*, 163t, 165, *165–166*

Electrocardiogram, interpretation of, 1–53
   step 1 (rhythm and rate), 1, *4*, *5*, *9*, 10, 10t
   step 2 (intervals and blocks), 10–16, *11–16*
   step 3 (atypical bundle branch block or WPW syndrome), 17, *17–19*
   step 4 (ST segment), 17, *19*, 20–24, *20–24*
   step 5 (Q waves), 24–34, *25–34*
   step 6 (P waves), 34, *35*, *36*
   step 7 (ventricular hypertrophy), *36*, 37, *37–39*
   step 8 (T waves), 37, *40–43*
   step 9 (electrical axis), 43, *44–45*, 46t
   step 10 (miscellaneous conditions), 47–51, *47*, 47t, *48–50*
   step 11 (arrhythmias), 51, 52
   normal, 3t, *4–8*
   technique of, 52, *52*, 53
   wave from of, *2*
Electrodes, misplacement of, *53*
   placement of, *52*
Electronic pacing, 183, 185–189
   atrial, 186, *186*
   atrioventricular, 186, *187*, *188*
   failure of, 189, *191–192*
   malfunction with, 189, *189–193*
   power failure during, 189, *193*
   undersensing malfunction of, 189, *189*, *190*
   ventricular, 183, 185, *185*
Emphysema, QS pattern in, 127, *130*

F

F wave, in atrial flutter, 234, *235*

H

Heart rate, assessment of, 10t
   in atrial fibrillation, 234
Hyperkalemia, *178*, 179
   QRS complex in, *178*, 179
   ST segment in, *178*, 179
   T wave in, *178*, 179
Hypokalemia, 176–179
   ST segment in, 176, *177*, 179
   T wave in, 176, *177*
   U wave in, 176, *177*, 179
Hypothermia, *195*, 196

I

Intraventricular conduction delay, assessment of, 17, *17, 19*

J

Junctional premature beats, 201, *201, 202*

K

Kawasaki disease, myocardial infarction and, 109, *122*

L

Leads, misplacement of, *52*
　placement of, *52*
Left anterior fascicular block, 166–170, *170*
　diagnostic criteria for, 167, *168, 170*
　right bundle branch block and, *169*
Left bundle branch block, 70–73
　causes of, 73
　diagnostic criteria for, *16*, 70, *70–73*
　myocardial infarction and, 131, *132, 133*
　QRS complex in, *11*, 14, *15–16, 16*, 70, *70, 71*
　R wave in, *16, 70–72*, 73, *73, 105*, 127
　ST segment elevation in, *72, 73*, 90
Left posterior fascicular block, *167*, 170–171, *170*
　right bundle branch block and, *170–171*
Left ventricular aneurysm, ST segment elevation in, *89*, 90

M

Mitral insufficiency, multifocal atrial tachycardia and, *226*
Multifocal atrial tachycardia, 225, *226*
Myocardial infarction, 106, 109–126
　age-indeterminate, *30*, 109, *120*
　anterior, Q wave in, 65, 109, *110–113*
　　assessment of, 24, *25, 28, 29*, 62
　　ST segment elevation in, *21*, 76, *80, 82–83, 89, 110–111*
　　vs. emphysema-related QS pattern, *130*
　anteroseptal, cocaine abuse and, *121*
　　Q wave in, 86, *87, 108*, 109, *114–115*

Myocardial infarction *(Continued)*
　　assessment of, 24, *25, 30*, 62
　　R wave in, 106, *108*
　　right bundle branch block and, 67
　　ST segment elevation in, 76, *79*, 86, *86*
　　vs. AIDS myocarditis, *126*
　　vs. left ventricular hypertrophy, *127*
　cocaine abuse and, 109, *121*
　diagnostic criteria for, *21*, 75–86, *75–87*, 106, 109, *111–120*
　inferior, cocaine abuse and, *121*
　　Q wave in, *25–27*, 67, 109, *116–117, 119*
　　ST segment elevation in, *20*, 76, *77, 78, 84–85, 116–117, 121*
　　vs. Wolff-Parkinson-White syndrome, 225, *227, 229*
　inferoposterior, Q wave in, *123*
　Kawasaki disease and, 109, *122*
　lateral, Q wave in, *25, 33*, 62, *120*
　left bundle branch block and, 131, *132, 133*
　mimics of, *16*, 126–127, *127, 128–130*
　non-Q-wave, ST segment depression in, *22*, 90, *91*
　　ST segment elevation in, 20, *22*
　posterior, Q wave in, 109
　　R wave in, 76, 109, *124*
　　ST segment elevation in, 76
　　T wave in, *124*
　Q wave persistence after, 109, *119*
　right bundle branch block and, 131
　right ventricular, Q wave in, 109, *123*
　　ST segment elevation in, 76, *84–85*
　size of, *82*, 86
　ST segment elevation in, 17, 20, *20–21, 20–22*, 75–86, *75–87*
Myocardial ischemia, ST segment depression in, *22*, 90, *92–96*
　ST segment elevation in, 20, *22, 23*
　T wave inversion in, 149, *150–153, 155–156*
　assessment of, 37, *40–43*
Myocarditis, AIDS, vs. anteroseptal myocardial infarction, *126*
　ST segment elevation in, 90
Myxedema, low-voltage QRS complex with, *134*, 135

N

Nodal premature beats, 201, *201, 202*

O

Orthodromic circus movement tachycardia, 230–231, *230, 231,* 232.
  See also *Wolff-Parkinson-White
  syndrome.*
Orthodromic tachycardia, 232. See
  also *Wolff-Parkinson-White
  syndrome.*
Osborn wave, in hypothermia, *195,* 196

P

P wave, abnormal, *35,* 54, *57, 58*
  absence of, 58
  assessment of, 34, *35, 36*
  diphasic, *35, 36,* 54, *57, 58*
  in atrioventricular junctional
    rhythm, 54, *57*
  in atrioventricular nodal reentrant
    tachycardia, 216, *219, 220,* 221,
    221
  in left atrial hypertrophy, *35,* 54, *57,*
    58, 136, *137*
  in multifocal atrial tachycardia, 58
  in paroxysmal atrial tachycardia,
    221–222, *222*
  in right atrial hypertrophy, *35, 36,*
    58, 137–138, *138*
  in right ventricular hypertrophy,
    143, 144
  in tachycardia, *219,* 219–221, *230,
    231,* 232
  in ventricular tachycardia, 238–239
  normal, *2,* 3t, *4,* 54, *55–56*
  premature, 197, *198–200*
Pacemaker rhythm, *49*
Paroxysmal atrial tachycardia,
    221–225, *222–224*
  with block, 222, *223, 224*
Pericarditis, *48,* 172–173
  electrical alternans in, 183, *184*
  ST segment in, *48,* 86, 87, 90, *174*
Persistent atrial tachycardia, 225
Pneumothorax, QS pattern in, 127
Postpericardiotomy syndrome, electri-
    cal alternans in, 183, *184*
PR interval, assessment of, 10, *11*
  in first-degree atrioventricular
    block, 209, *209*
  in second-degree atrioventricular
    block, 210, *211*

PR interval *(Continued)*
  normal, 3t
  of atrial premature beat, 197
PR segment, in pericarditis, 173
Prolonged QT interval, 174–176, *175,
    176*
  causes of, 176
Pseudo-Q wave, in Wolff-Parkinson-
    White syndrome, 127, *128*
Pulmonary embolism, 189, *194,* 196
  QS pattern in, 127
  ST segment elevation in, 90, *194*

Q

Q wave, 61–63, *62,* 98–135. See also *R
    wave, loss of.*
  assessment of, 24–34, *25–34,* 98,
    99. See also *R wave, loss of.*
  depth of, *100, 102,* 102–103
  in AIDS myocarditis, *126,* 127
  in anterior myocardial infarction,
    24, *25,* 28, *29, 62,* 65, 109,
    110–113
  in anteroseptal myocardial infarc-
    tion, 24, *25, 30, 62,* 86, *87,
    108,* 109, *114–115*
  in chest trauma, 127
  in emphysema, 127, *130*
  in hypertrophic cardiomyopathy, 63,
    126–127, 127
  in inferior myocardial infarction,
    25–27, 67, 109, *116–117, 119*
  in inferoposterior myocardial infarc-
    tion, *123*
  in lateral myocardial infarction, *25,
    33, 62, 120*
  in left bundle branch block, 131,
    132, 133
  in myocardial infarction, 106, 109,
    111–120
  in pneumothorax, 127
  in posterior myocardial infarction,
    109
  in pulmonary embolism, 127
  in right bundle branch block, 131
  in right ventricular infarction, 109,
    123
  narrow, *7, 62, 100,* 102
  nondiagnostic changes in, *118*
  normal, 3t, *5, 7,* 10t, *62, 62,*
    98–103, *99–104*
  small, *5, 62, 62, 101,* 102, *103, 118*
  technical error and, *53,* 63

QR complex, in ventricular tachycardia, 238, *239*
QRS complex, 59–63
  alternans of, 183
  assessment of, 10, *11, 12*
  in hyperkalemia, *178,* 179
  in left bundle branch block, *11,* 14, *15–16,* 70, *70, 71*
  in left ventricular hypertrophy, *139*
  in paroxysmal atrial tachycardia, *222–224,* 225
  in right bundle branch block, 10, *11–14, 13,* 60, 64–65, *65–67*
  in third-degree atrioventricular block, 210, *214, 215*
  in ventricular tachycardia, 238, *239–242*
  low-voltage, 131, *134,* 135
  negative, 63
  normal, 3t, 61, *62*
  rotation-related variation in, 24, *28,* 61, *62*
  vector forces of, 59–61, *60*
QRS vector, 160, *160*
QT interval, assessment of, 47, 47t
  corrected, 175
  normal, 47t
  prolongation of, 174–176, *175, 176*
    causes of, 176
  short, 176

R
R wave, 59, 60, *60*
  height of, 61
  in left bundle branch block, *16, 70–72,* 73, *73, 105,* 127
  in posterior myocardial infarction, 76, 109, *124*
  in right bundle branch block, *13,* 64, *65, 66*
  in Wolff-Parkinson-White syndrome, 17, *17,* 17t, *18*
  late transition of, 24, *25, 34,* 106, *106*
  loss of, *99*
    assessment of, 24–34, *25–34*
    in anterior myocardial infarction, *21,* 24, *25, 28, 29, 31, 32,* 62
    in anteroseptal myocardial infarction, 24, *25, 30,* 62
    in inferior myocardial infarction, 24, *26–27*
    in lateral myocardial infarction, *25, 33,* 62, *120*

R wave *(Continued)*
  normal, 3t
  poor progression of, 86, *99,* 103, *104–106*
    assessment of, 24, *25, 34*
    in anteroseptal myocardial infarction, 106, *108*
    normal, *104, 106*
  tall, 17t, *37, 38,* 61
Rhythm, assessment of, 1, *4, 5, 9*
Right bundle branch block, 64–69
  causes of, 65
  diagnostic criteria for, 64, *65–67*
  incomplete, *49,* 67, *68*
  left anterior fascicular block and, *169*
  left posterior fascicular block and, *170–171*
  myocardial infarction and, 65, 67, 131
  QRS complex in, *60,* 64–65, *65–67*
    assessment of, 10, *11–14*
  R wave in, *13,* 64, *65, 66*
  S wave in, *13,* 64, *65, 66,* 67, *68*
Romhilt-Estes scoring system, for left ventricular hypertrophy, 141
RR interval, in second-degree atrioventricular block, 210, *211, 212*
RS interval, in ventricular tachycardia, 238
RSr′ variant, 67, *68,* 69, *69*
  in atrial septal defect, *49,* 69

S
S wave, 60, *60*
  in right bundle branch block, *13,* 64, *65, 66,* 67, *68*
Sinus rhythm, 1, *5*
Sinus tachycardia, 216, *218*
Sokolow-Lyon voltage criteria, for left ventricular hypertrophy, *37,* 139, *140,* 141
ST segment, *2,* 74–97
  assessment of, 17, *19,* 20–24, *20–24,* 74, *75*
  depression of, in acute myocardial infarction, 76
    in hypokalemia, 176, *177,* 179
    in myocardial ischemia, *22,* 90, *92–96*
    in non-Q-wave myocardial infarction, *22,* 90, *91*

ST segment (*Continued*)
  elevation of, 17, *19*, 20, *20*, *21*, 74
    fishhook appearance of, *24*, 76, 87, *88*
    in acute myocardial infarction, 75–86, *75–87*
    in age-indeterminate myocardial infarction, *30*, 90
    in anterior myocardial infarction, *21*, 76, 80, *82–83*, 89, *110–111*
    in anteroseptal myocardial infarction, 76, *79*, 86, *86*
    in athlete, *88*
    in cocaine abuse, 90
    in coronary artery spasm, 90
    in hyperkalemia, *178*, 179
    in hypertrophic cardiomyopathy, 90
    in inferior myocardial infarction, *20*, 76, *77*, *78*, *84–85*, *116–117*, *121*
    in left bundle branch block, *72*, *73*, 90
    in left ventricular aneurysm, *89*, 90
    in left ventricular hypertrophy, *36*, *37*, 90
    in myocardial ischemia, 20, *22*, *23*
    in myocarditis, 90
    in non-Q-wave myocardial infarction, 20, *22*
    in pericarditis, 87, 90, *174*
    in posterior myocardial infarction, 76
    in pulmonary embolism, 90, *194*
    in Q wave myocardial infarction, 17, 20, *20–21*
    in right ventricular infarction, 76, *84–85*
    normal, 20, *24*, 76, 87, *88*
    variation in, *81*
  in pericarditis, *48*, 86
  isoelectric, in anterolateral infarction, *120*
    in inferior infarction, *119*
  nonspecific changes in, 96–97, *96*, *97*
  normal, *3t*, 96
  ST-T wave, in acute myocardial infarction, 86, *87*
Subarachnoid hemorrhage, T wave inversion in, 149, *157*
Supraventricular tachycardia, *219*, *220*

T
T wave, 145–159
  assessment of, 37, *40–43*, 145, *146–148*
  diphasic, 54
  in atrial trigeminy, *200*
  in hyperkalemia, *178*, 179
  in hypokalemia, 176, *177*
  in hypothermia, *195*, 196
  in myocardial ischemia, 37, *40–43*, 149, *150–153*, *155–156*
  in pericarditis, 173
  in posterior myocardial infarction, *124*
  in pulmonary embolism, *194*
  in subarachnoid hemorrhage, 149, *157*
  inversion of, *43*, 145, 149, *150–157*
    minor, *149*, 158–159
    symmetric, 149
  nonspecific changes in, *154*
  normal, 3t, 145, *148*, *149*
  repolarization changes in, 159
  tall, *158*, 159
Tachycardia, 216–247, *217*
  antidromic circus movement, *245*. See also *Wolff-Parkinson-White syndrome.*
  atrial, multifocal, 225, *226*
    persistent, 225
  carotid sinus massage in, 232
  IV adenosine in, 232
  narrow QRS, 216–234, *217–224*, *226–231*, *233*, *235–237*. See also specific types.
    assessment of, *51*, 52
    differential diagnosis of, 231–232
  orthodromic circus movement, 230–231, *231*
  P wave in, *219*, *219–221*, 230, *230*, *231*, 232
  sinus, 216, *218*
  wide QRS, *217*, 234–247
    assessment of, *51*, 52
    irregular, 239, *244*, *245*, *246–247*
    regular, 234, 238–239, *239–242*. See also *Ventricular tachycardia.*
Torsades de pointes, 246–247, *246*

U
U wave, in hypokalemia, 176, *177*, 179

V

Ventricular bigeminy, *205*
Ventricular hypertrophy, left, 139–141,
    141
    assessment of, *36, 37, 37*
    Cornell voltage criteria for, 141
    diagnostic criteria for, *37,* 139,
        140, 141
    QRS complex in, *139*
    R wave in, *37,* 61
    Romhilt-Estes scoring system for,
        141
    Sokolow-Lyon voltage criteria for,
        37, 139, *140,* 141
    ST segment elevation in, *36, 37,*
        90
    vs. left bundle branch block, 73
  right, 141, *143,* 144
    assessment of, *36, 37, 38–39*
    diagnostic criteria for, 141, 144,
        144
    P wave in, *143,* 144
    R wave in, 17t, *38,* 61
Ventricular premature beats, 201–206,
    203–208

Ventricular premature beats *(Continued)*
  couplets of, 206, *206, 208*
  multifocal, 206, *208*
  salvos of, 206, *206, 208*
  unifocal, 206
Ventricular tachycardia, 234, 238–239,
    239–242
  nonsustained, 206, *207,* 208
  QRS complex in, 238, *239–242*
  sinus rhythm and, *242*

W

Wolff-Parkinson-White syndrome, 225,
    227–229, 230–232, *231, 245*
  antidromic tachycardia in, *244*
  assessment of, 17, *17,* 17t, *18*
  delta wave in, 225, *227–228*
  electrical alternans in, 183, *184*
  pseudo-Q wave in, 127, *128*
  R wave in, 17, *17,* 17t, *18*
  type A, 225, *227–228*
  type B, 225, *228*
  types of, 232
  vs. inferior myocardial infarction,
    225, *227, 229*